THE CANCER INDUSTRY

CRIMES, CONSPIRACY AND THE DEATH OF MY MOTHER

MARK SLOAN

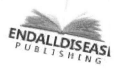

ENDALLDISEASE
PUBLISHING

D0905834

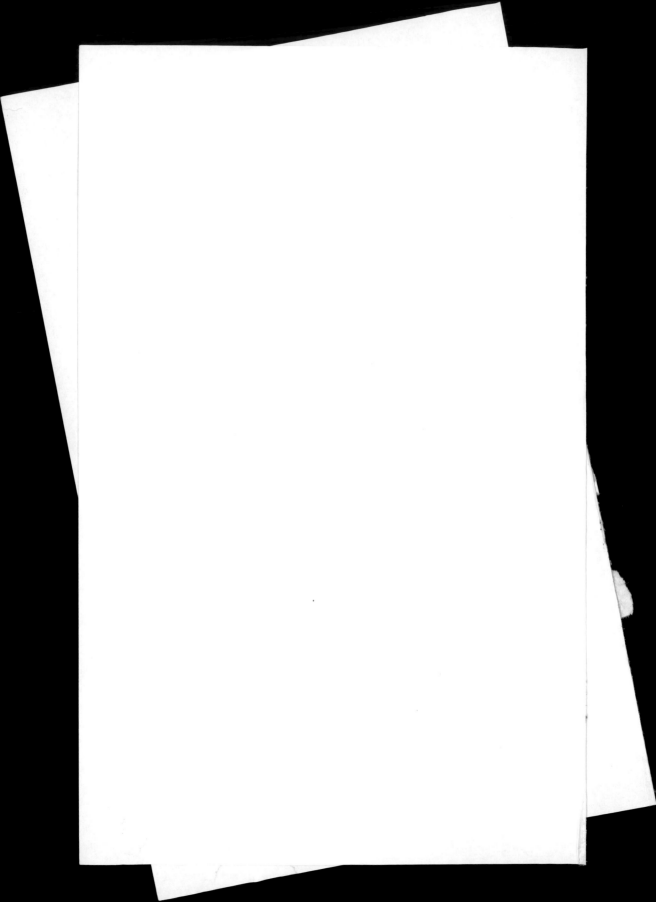

Contents

ACKNOWLEDGEMENTS	I
PREFACE	1
INTRODUCTION	9

SURGERY	13
HISTORY OF CANCER SURGERY	14
FOUR SHOCKING CANCER SURGERIES	15
A MESSAGE FROM DR. IAN HARRIS	18
MILLIONS OF POINTLESS OPERATIONS EVERY YEAR	19
CORONARY ARTERY BYPASS SURGERY	20
SURGERY VS. CANCER	22
CANCER SURGERY PROMOTES METASTASIS	23
THE STRESS OF SURGERY	25
16 WAYS SURGERY CAUSES CANCER	29
TIMELESS QUOTES	33

CHEMOTHERAPY	35
FROM BATTLEFIELD TO CANCER CLINIC	36
CHEMOTHERAPY VS. CANCER	38
SUCCESS STORIES?	40
ADDITIONAL HEALTH EFFECTS	41
TIMELESS QUOTES	48

RADIOTHERAPY	51
THE DISCOVERY OF X-RAYS	52
SHOE-FITTING X-RAY FLUOROSCOPES	52
FLUOROSCOPES AS ENTERTAINMENT	53

RADIOTHERAPY VS. CANCER 53
RADIOTHERAPY ADMINISTERS 5X THE FATAL DOSE 54
WHISTLEBLOWER EXPOSES CANCER MORTALITY STATISTICS 57
RADIOTHERAPY ELEVATES LIFETIME RISK OF CANCER 58
RADIATION BYSTANDER EFFECTS......................................60
SUCCESS STORIES? 63
ADDITIONAL HEALTH EFFECTS..64
TIMELESS QUOTES 70

EARLY DETECTION, EARLY CURE?   71

THE PSA TEST: PROSTATE CANCER SCREENING 72
MAMMOGRAPHY: BREAST CANCER SCREENING 78
CANCER SCREENING: A PUBLIC HEALTH DISASTER 86
TIMELESS QUOTES 88

THE BATTLE FOR TRUTH   89

THE PSYCHOLOGY OF THE RICH 90
THE CANCER INDUSTRY'S BAG OF TRICKS 90
THE BATTLE FOR TRUTH..97
MANY 'CANCERS' NOT EVEN HARMFUL...................................99
SPONTANEOUS REGRESSION OF CANCER 103
THE CANCER INDUSTRY'S BIGGEST SECRET 105
TIMELESS QUOTES 108

CONCLUSION   109
REFERENCES   113
INDEX   189
ABOUT THE AUTHOR   195

ACKNOWLEDGEMENTS

Although the research and writing that went into this book amounted to a few thousand hours of my time and many hardships, in no way would it have been possible without the life's work of Dr. Raymond Peat. For a life devoted to courageously exploring the unknown in search of empirical truth, and for preserving, consolidating and advancing the quintessential observations reported by a number of maverick scientists over the past 150 years and then freely sharing your interpretations with the world - it's time that your work be known and understood by all. Your guidance and generosity in responding to the many questions I had during the writing process of this book have been instrumental.

Many thanks also to a number of other independent researchers for sharing your thoughts and ideas along the way.

Last but not least, I'd like to thank my father for putting up with me all these years; and also for handing down the work ethic, discipline and fortitude that was needed to complete this work.

PREFACE

"...I don't think she knew it at the time but I could hear every sob, every whimper and every call out to God to put an end to her suffering."

My entrance into this world came on mother's day in the spring of 1985 – and it came in epic fashion. With my mother's umbilical cord wrapped tightly around my neck, nurses and doctors scrambled to free me from my umbilical neuse before it was too late. I can only imagine how my parents must have felt as they watched the doctor yank me out of the womb and scramble to uncoil the cord from my neck. Fortunately, the efforts of the medical personnel paid off and my mother and father had a brand new son.

Growing up in Ontario, Canada with my parents and sister was not unlike that of your typical two-child family, but we were unique in some ways. One of the things that separated us from the herd was that my father ran his own business, which he started from scratch after finding out he and my mother had their first baby on the way. He knew the job he had couldn't provide the life he wanted for his family, so he risked everything and made it happen. While working day and night trying to build a successful business, my mother spent her time cooking, cleaning and taking care of my sister and I at home.

I had a great set of friends. I remember playing street hockey with them like it was yesterday. After putting down the sticks we would play tag, swim, light fires and most days you could find me riding my 3-wheel 'big wheelie' bike. In winter, we would carve tunnels into the mountain of snow piled high at the top of our street and *whiz* snowballs at each other. Aside from having to wake up early to attend school and the uncomfortable reality that success in school seemed to be about mindlessly repeating what we were told, things were going well. But as we all learn eventually, life is fragile, and things can change in an instant.

On a cold morning in grade 7, my father sat my sister and I down on the couch in the living room and told us he had an announcement to make. Although I was hoping to hear about an upcoming family vacation somewhere warm, I knew by his expression that the news was not going to be good.

He told us our mother had cancer.

The cancer was on her cervix and only about the size of a baby fingernail; and although I didn't know much about cancer at the time, hearing that doctors had detected it early and were going to rush her in for surgery and radiation made me feel hopeful.

Then our father told us it was too much for him to run a business and be a father and a mother to us at the same time, so he was flying in our aunt Kim from Alberta to help out for a number of months while mom recovered. My sister and I were both big fans of our aunt Kim and uncle Bob from out west, so we felt like we had just won the lottery.

Following surgery and radiation treatments, doctors assured us they 'got it all' and that my mother was cancer-free. My father wanted to make sure the cancer wasn't going to return so he took her to the best naturopathic doctor he knew, who put her on a number of dietary supplements. My father also did some research of his own and discovered Essiac - the famous 4-herb tea blend that nurse Renee Caisse of Bracebridge, Ontario had used to allegedly cure cancer patients for about 50 years until her death in 1978. He ordered the herbs and brewed them carefully following the instructions and administered it to my mother a number of times.

Unfortunately, after my mother's surgical and radiation therapy treatments, cutbacks at the hospital prevented us from having follow-up testing done. Eight months later, when we were finally able to have doctors run some follow-up tests, they encountered an aggressive cancer in her hip area: doctor's recommended chemotherapy and more radiation. Feeling afraid and out of options, we rushed her in for treatment once again.

The dramatic decline of her health following chemotherapy and radiotherapy treatments was obvious. I remember lying in bed late at night at the age of 11, hearing her pace back and forth in the living room below, struggling not to cry so we could sleep undisturbed. I don't think she knew it at the time but I could hear every sob, every whimper and every call out to God to put an end to her suffering.

Why was my mother in pain? I thought we had some of the best doctors in the country using the best treatments available, yet everything the doctors had done just seemed to make things worse. I felt angry and confused.

After a few long and difficult months, I woke up one morning to a scene in my living room that I will never forget: with tears rolling down his cheeks, my father sat my sister and I down on the couch next to aunt Kim and told us our mother was gone. I felt shocked and overwhelmed. I remember holding my breath to try and avoid feeling the intense emotions welling up inside me.

Dad spoke about the scene in the hospital earlier that morning right before our mother had died. Together with her mother and father, her five brothers and sisters and a priest from our local church, they formed a circle around her hospital bed and prayed. Aunt Kim told us the presence she felt in the room during those last moments was unlike anything she had experienced before. Dad agreed. While laying on the hospital bed, the very last thing my mother did - just seconds before exhaling her final breath - was lift her arms straight up towards the heavens above to be received by God.

Losing my mother was like losing my biggest fan; it was the ultimate setback in my development growing up, and it happened at the worst possible time - right before starting high school. What's worse, every time I was around people I felt like my emotions needed to be kept secret; like I needed to pretend that I was okay, and that if anybody ever truly understood how I felt, they wouldn't want to be around me because it would be too uncomfortable for them.

My family and I tried counseling, but I knew the therapist was only there because he was getting paid, so it ended up making me feel even angrier. I needed my mother - not some imposter pretending to care. My bottled up emotions had no place to go, so inside they remained. I accepted an award for *diligence and determination* at grade 8 graduation and moved on to highschool.

At highschool, I spent most of my time in the weight room; every lunch, every break, and sometimes I would even skip class to workout. I loved it in there! I felt like once again I had a group of friends I could trust; friends who shared a similar interest in fitness and were striving to become something better. Strength training provided me with the opportunity to continually challenge myself and break through my own limitations. It was in the gym where I first discovered that although there were plenty of guys who were bigger than me, none of them could outwork me. I remember in grade 11, weighing just 160lbs, my record shoulder press was 110lbs in each hand for 8 reps.

But far more than any muscle or strength I happened to gain, the weight room was the first place I had known where it was both safe and beneficial for me to express my anger. Finally I had found a way to channel the throbbing stockpile of emotions inside me into something useful; something that would benefit me and perhaps inspire others.

After graduating high school, I went on to college and earned a diploma in Fire Sciences. Along the way I learned a few things: First, very little of what was taught in the course was actually useful for preparing me to work as a firefighter. Somehow going into a 100% concrete structure with fire gear on and spraying water onto a steel crate of burning wood doesn't quite capture the reality of a fire scene. Secondly, even though I had the fastest time running up and down stairs with a hose on my back during tryouts for the *Firefighter Combat Challenge*, I learned that firefighting is a political man's game - and since I don't play games, someone slower got the spot on the team instead. Last but not least, the most valuable lessons in college are learned outside of class. In my final year, one of my roommates showed me a documentary that made me question my entire reality and the world around me. I wasn't sure if the information was true or not, but I knew I had to find out.

From an early age I had been drawn towards books on self-help and nutrition. I loved the fact that I could read about different theories and then test them myself to see what worked and what didn't. Constant and never-ending improvement was the path I was on from the beginning and I never had any doubt that I could change the world or accomplish whatever I wanted to in life.

With the age of the internet in full swing, suddenly I found myself on a quest for truth; broadening my horizons and obsessively exploring all avenues of research I could find - in books, articles and documentaries - for 8, 10, sometimes 12 hours or more per day. I also spent a lot of time integrating this newfound knowledge into my own articles and documentaries, then sharing my work with whoever was interested through my website and the power of social media. Almost 10 years after my search for truth began - it hit me.

I realized that my mother's death was not a tragedy, but an opportunity. She gave me a story to tell that could move people and a mind that could find the answers the world was literally dying to know; I realized that my mother died so my life could have purpose.

In return for this gift, I made a promise to her in my heart that I would solve the riddle of cancer so that no child would have to go through what I did, ever again. I knew that once I found the answers and shared them with the world, the legacy of my mother would transform from a victim of cancer to a hero who inspired her son to save lives and change the world.

INTRODUCTION

IT'S BEEN NEARLY 50 years since the *War on Cancer* was declared, and yet more people are diagnosed with cancer and dying from the disease than ever before.[1]

I find it extraordinarily difficult to believe that after spending $500 billion dollars on cancer research since 1970,[2] the cancer establishment has come up with literally nothing useful for preventing or curing the disease. If it's true, then they are incompetent and their astonishing lack of advancement is undoubtedly the most spectacular failure in human history. But if cures or effective treatments have been systematically suppressed from the public, then their actions are criminal in nature and blood from over 530 million people[3] could be on their hands. Whatever the case may be, I intend to make it clear.

Up until this point on humankind's pursuit to end cancer, our primary mistake has been entrusting the same people who profit from treating cancer to provide us with a cure. I haven't spoken to anyone who didn't understand this concept - there is no money in a cure. Why would an industry that generates over $125 billion dollars a year[4] put itself out of business? It wouldn't.

So who then do we look to for answers?

In 1947, the young American physicist Ernest Sternglass wrote a letter to Albert Einstein telling him about the work he had been doing to reduce radiation doses during X-ray fluoroscopy. To his surprise, Einstein showed great interest in his work and invited the 23-year-old to meet with him at Princeton University, where they talked for 5 hours. "And that had an enormous effect on my life. Because among other things, he encouraged me to pursue my theory and I finally got it all published," recalls Sternglass.[5]

At the end of their conversation, Einstein issued a very important warning: "Don't go back into academia," he said. "They will kill every bit of originality out of you. In order to become a full professor, you have to get approved on every level and you cannot question the existing ideas too much or else you won't get promoted... have a shoemaker's job for the rest of your life, so that you can do something useful for humanity."

My purpose in writing this book is to explore the possibility that, hidden somewhere inside the digital trash heap known as the internet, the disease of cancer has already been solved. And while a doctor might fear losing his medical license or job for completing such work, a layperson with no medical background like myself can fearlessly make a controversial conclusion when the evidence warrants one. This pure and unobstructed curiosity combined with discipline and an intention to simplify complex information will render a final product on the cutting edge of science that can be understood by those who need it.

FOR THE TIME IS AT HAND

The American Cancer Society estimates that almost half of everybody alive today will develop cancer at some point in their lives,[6] and the World Health Organization predicts a 50% rise in cancer diagnosis' by the year 2020.[7]

Unless we figure out what is fuelling this explosion of cancer rates and alter our course, a time will soon come when nobody escapes the ravages of this disease. The future of human civilization is at stake and only one thing is certain - if the answers are out there, they will be found.

CHAPTER 1

SURGERY

A SURGEON'S FIRST instinct when he sees a patient with a tumor is to reach for his scalpel and carve it out of them. This makes it easy to assume patients are benefitting from this kind of treatment, but removal of a tumor isn't simply a local phenomenon with no other biological consequences.

Although surgical removal of a tumor is widely accepted today as beneficial and necessary, it was not long ago that the prevailing public attitude towards tumor resection (and other cancer treatments used today) was so disapproving and hostile that it can be difficult for people to imagine. "It should be forbidden and severely punished to remove cancer by cutting, burning, cautery and other fiendish tortures," wrote 15th century renaissance physician Paracelsus.

Whether you've been cut by a criminal in the street because you refused to give him your wallet, or by a surgeon on an operating table because you gave him your wallet, the act of cutting into the body is traumatic and inflicts damage.

In this chapter we will investigate the impact of surgery on health and determine if tumor removal is beneficial for a person with cancer. But first, a little history on the subject of cancer surgery.

HISTORY OF CANCER SURGERY

The rapid rise of cancer surgery is best illustrated by the early history of what is now called the Memorial Sloan-Kettering Cancer Center in New York, wrote Dr. Ralph Moss in his book *The Cancer Industry.*

A 19th century "Women's doctor" named J. Marion Sims was the spiritual founder of the Memorial Sloan-Kettering Cancer Center. Sims received a very brief medical training before he began performing surgery. While some tattoo artists develop their skills by practicing on the skin of pigs or even the porous skin of a grapefruit, Sims began his training on a group of slave women from the southern United States. In a makeshift 'hospital' behind his house, Sims began dozens of experimental procedures on the women. Some of these women received as many as thirty operations in a four-year period.

According to his biographer, these operations were said to be "little short of murderous."

After he felt he was ready to move on, Sims moved to New York City where he founded Women's Hospital, which still exists to this day. Sims developed a select clientele of wealthy women and European immigrants upon which he continued to perform large numbers of surgeries.

According to Dr. Moss, The Lady Managers (trustees) of the hospital became convinced that "the lives of all the patients in the institution were being threatened by… mysterious experiments." Sims was expelled from the hospital, but was then reinstated a short time later.

In 1884, Sims went on to establish the first private cancer hospital in the United States, The New York Cancer Hospital, known today as the Memorial Sloan-Kettering Cancer Center. Sims was set to become the first director of the hospital, but he died before he had a chance to fill the position.

FOUR SHOCKING CANCER SURGERIES

If you found the history of cancer surgery itself shocking, wait until you learn about 4 of the most grotesque cancer surgeries of the past. The four surgeries we're going to look at now are called *The Commando*, *The Whipple*, *Total Exenteration* and the *Hemicorporectomy*.

The Commando

The Commando was performed on patients who had been diagnosed with tongue cancer and involved the surgical removal of a patient's entire mandible or jaw. Could you imagine living life after having literally half your face removed?

According to one surgeon, The Commando "derived its wide acceptance from the fact that it brought to mind the slashing attack of the world war I commandos" (Crile, 1974).

The Whipple

The Whipple was type of cancer surgery developed for the treatment of pancreatic cancer by president of the American Surgical Association and clinical director at Memorial hospital, Dr. Allen Oldfather Whipple.

This ghastly surgery involved the removal of many organs adjacent to the affected gland, on the theory that they might be harboring nests of cancer cells (National Cancer Institute, 1976).

Total Exenteration

In 1948, Dr. Alexander Brunshwig from Memorial Hospital invented an operation called Total Exenteration.

Total Exenteration involved the removal of all of the following organs and internal body parts:

- The rectum
- The stomach
- The bladder
- Part of the liver
- The ureter
- All internal reproductive organs
- The pelvic floor and wall
- The pancreas
- The spleen
- The colon
- Many blood vessels

In an article in the New York Times dated April 8th, 1969, Dr. Brunschwig himself called the operation "A brutal and cruel procedure."

THE HEMICORPORECTOMY

Last but certainly not the least in our list of four cruel and brutal cancer procedures is The Hemicorporectomy. This surgery involved literally, the removal of half the body.

The Hemicorporectomy was developed by Dr. Theodore Miller - another Memorial Hospital surgeon - for the treatment of bladder or pelvic malignancy. This surgery involved the amputation of everything below the pelvis. Not surprisingly, many patients chose death over submitting to Miller's operation (New York Times, November 30, 1969).

The most astounding thing about the four surgeries we just covered is this:

<u>All of them are still being peformed to this day.</u> Yes, every single surgery just mentioned are still on the menu for surgeons. None have been banned. Look them up and you will find recent articles of various people undergoing them in recent years. A cancer surgeon can (and may) recommend any of these surgeries if you consult him or her.

A MESSAGE FROM DR. IAN HARRIS

I realize this is a bit of a digression but it's important and will provide you with some solace following that heavily disturbing information before we go on.

In 2018 I had the pleasure of interviewing Australian Surgeon Dr. Ian Harris, author of the book *Surgery: The Ultimate Placebo*. At the end of the interview, I asked him his most important message that he'd like everybody in the world to know, and he said:

"The effectiveness of medicine is overestimated by those who are making the decisions and the harms are underestimated. The doctors that sell are overestimating the benefits and underestimating the harms. The way to correct that is to make doctors be more scientific about what they do, and also to educate the public to be more scientific about what they will have done to them. Don't be afraid to look up the evidence. Ask your doctor questions. The simplest question of all, and it sounds dumb but so many unnecessary procedures could've been saved by asking this single question: What evidence do you have that doing this procedure to me is better than not doing it to me?"

MILLIONS OF POINTLESS OPERATIONS EVERY YEAR

Common sense tells us that if a surgical procedure isn't needed then it shouldn't be performed. Nevertheless, some studies estimate that as many as 30% of certain surgeries are performed unnecessarily,[1] and some claim the numbers are actually much, much higher.

A 1995 report by Milliman & Robertson, Inc. concluded that nearly 60 percent of all surgeries performed are medically unnecessary,[2] but even that number is considered low by the late American pediatrician Dr. Robert Mendelsohn who wrote, "My feeling is that somewhere around ninety percent of surgery is a waste of time, energy, money, and life."[3]

Research on unnecessary surgery began in 1974, after a US congressional report estimated that 2.4 million unnecessary surgeries were performed every year, killing nearly 12,000 patients.[4] This report caught the eye of Harvard professor and former surgeon Lucian Leape, who has been following this line of research ever since.

Leape's take today? "Things haven't changed very much."[5]

A 2016 review of the latest research on unnecessary surgery states, "Worldwide every year millions of patients go under knife, but many of them are enduring great pain and shelling out thousands and dollars for surgeries they don't really need."[6]

Not only are many people put 'under the knife' needlessly, but Australia's top surgeon Dr. Ian Harris says that many commonly-performed operations of today "are no better than placebo."[7] In his new book *Surgery, The Ultimate Placebo*, Dr. Harris lists a number of "placebo surgeries," including spinal fusion for back pain, knee arthroscopy, coronary stenting, some shoulder surgery and appendix removal, laparoscopy for bowel adhesions and repairs of ruptured tendons and some fractures.

CORONARY ARTERY BYPASS SURGERY

One of the most common and expensive surgeries performed in America today is the coronary artery bypass - a procedure that grafts a new vein in place of a damaged one supplying the heart. According to Dr. Mark Hyman and Dr. Mark Liponis in their book *Ultraprevention*, "Bypasses are the single most commonly performed unnecessary surgery in the country." I reviewed the scientific literature to find out if there was any support for this claim, and the evidence seems to agree.[8-10]

A CLOSER LOOK...

The first ever clinical trial on coronary artery bypass surgery was published in The Lancet in 1977 and compared heart disease patients who underwent bypass surgery with ones who received drug treatment only. Results showed that survival at four years was 3% lower in those who underwent surgery.[8]

In the Coronary Artery Bypass Study of 1984, 780 heart disease patients were randomly assigned either surgical or drug treatments and evaluated 5-years later. "The five-year probability of remaining alive and free of infarction [heart attack] was 82 per cent in the patients assigned to medical therapy and 83 per cent in the patients assigned to surgery (not significant)."[9]

A 1999 study from the journal *Circulation* compared the effectiveness of coronary angioplasty, coronary artery bypass surgery and drug treatment on heart disease patients. After a 5-year follow-up, researchers found that all three treatments "yielded a similar incidence of acute myocardial infarction and death."[10]

Despite clear evidence showing that cardiac bypass surgery provides no benefit to patients, more than 200,000 procedures are performed every year in the United States.[11] A 2016 study published in *The American Journal of Cardiology* asked 101 US hospitals what they charge for coronary artery bypass surgery, and of the 53 hospitals that responded, the average cost for the procedure was $151,271, ranging from $44,824 to $448,038. Buyer beware: the study found "no evidence to suggest that hospitals that charge higher prices provide better quality of care."[12]

As it turns out, cracking open people's chests and dicing up their arteries remains a treasured source of income for surgeons, while patients end up broke and no healthier than they were before the procedure. And considering coronary artery bypass surgery comes with serious potential complications like impotence,[13] brain damage, organ dysfunction,[14] or even death, the evidence suggests far more harm is being done than good.

Now, how about cancer surgery?

SURGERY VS. CANCER

The most comprehensive study ever undertaken on the efficacy of cancer surgery, to date, was conducted in 1844 by Dr. Leroy d'Etoilles of Paris, France and published in *The French Academy of Science*. After studying 2,781 cancer patients over a 30-year period who had undergone either surgery, caustics (application of a chemical that destroys tissue) or no treatment at all, Dr. d'Etoilles found that the average survival of patients following surgery was one year and five months. Remarkably, two years after cancer diagnosis, those who refused both surgery and caustics had a 50% higher rate of survival.[15]

Recent research has validated Dr. d'Etoilles pioneering work, showing that cutting out a tumor either provides no benefit to patients,[16,18] or increases mortality.[17,143,144] The more the body is cut, the worse the outcome appears to be.

CANCER SURGERY PROMOTES METASTASIS

Cancer metastasis is the primary cause of most cancer deaths,[20-22] and yet the public remains almost completely unaware that surgical removal of a tumor has been known to cause cancer metastasis for over 100 years.

In 1910, researchers implanted tumors into mice and found when they left the tumors alone, cancer metastasis almost never occurred. But when they incompletely cut out the tumors, metastasis frequently occurred.[23] A few years later a similar experiment was conducted using highly metastasizing tumors, and the results were the same - tumor resection increased cancer metastasis compared to control mice whose tumors were left untouched.[24]

This same phenomenon was demonstrated in humans by Dr. Warren Cole of the University of Illinois in 1974. In a series of experiments published in the *Annals of the New York Academy of Sciences,* Dr. Cole wrote, "Ten of our patients underwent an unsuccessful attempt by a surgeon to remove the tumor. All surgeons know that this procedure is usually followed by an increased growth of the tumor...metastasis develops so commonly after excision of the primary."[25]

German professor of Radiology Dr. Ernst H. Krokowski provided further evidence that surgery, and even tumor palpation and biopsy promote the spread of cancer. In a 1979 study, Dr. Krokowski wrote, "... manipulation of the tumor, such as severe palpation, biopsy or surgery, results in a sudden increase of the number of tumor cells released into the blood circulation."

Dr. Krokowski also stated that about 90% of patients die from metastasis or secondary tumors and "Therefore it should be of great concern to therapists as well as patients that already more than 30 years ago it was conclusively shown that cancer surgery is the main cause of metastasis. However, this research was completely ignored by the profession, it was just too awful to contemplate, and patients never got to know about it."[26]

Since 1996, Dr. Michael Retsky of Harvard University and his international team of colleagues have been investigating the physiological mechanisms behind surgically-induced cancer metastasis. In a 2010 review of their work, they stated that tumors aren't in continuous growth as it was once thought. Instead, they undergo periods of dormancy, where they are sitting harmlessly and "surgery to remove the primary tumor often terminates dormancy resulting in accelerated relapses."[27]

Studies worldwide have demonstrated consistently and repeatedly that surgical removal of a tumor often terminates dormancy and leads to cancer metastasis.[28-34] Furthermore, surgical removal of lymph nodes (lymphadenectomy), which is standard practice following tumor removal for breast and skin cancer, was found in 2015 to increase "the growth of the primary tumor and associated blood vessels as well as promoted cancer cell survival and dissemination."[19]

Even the former director of the National Cancer Institute Vincent J. Davita Jr. wrote about surgically-induced cancer metastasis in the world's definitive, standard-setting oncology textbook *Cancer: Principles and*

Practise of Oncology in 1982. "There seems to be little doubt that cancer can be spread from the primary site to distant tissues. There are numerous ways that surgical manipulation could be responsible for this."

THE STRESS OF SURGERY

Few people but surgeons are aware that the stress induced by surgery can result in serious, potentially fatal complications. Like all forms of stress, surgery activates the sympathetic 'flight or fight' nervous system,[35] which elevates stress hormones to liberate glucose from the liver and breakdown fat and muscle as additional energy sources to meet the demands of the upcoming fight.[36]

Even when a surgeon performs an operation successfully with no errors, the stress caused by being cut in one area of the body can lead to damage in another. Complications of surgical stress include, but are not limited to:

Blood Health:

- Surgical stress causes a loss of blood albumin[37]

Bone Health:

- Surgical stress causes bone loss (osteoporosis)[38,39]

Brain Health:

- Surgical stress causes delirium[40]

- Surgical stress causes cognitive dysfunction[41]

- Surgical stress causes memory impairment[42,78]

- Surgical stress causes nerve damage[44]

- Surgical stress causes stroke[45]

- Surgical stress causes seizures[46]

- Surgical stress causes paralysis[47]

Dental Health:

- Surgical stress causes dental caries (cavities)[48]

Depression:

- Surgical stress causes anxiety and depression[43,49]

Diabetes:

- Surgical stress causes insulin-resistance[50]

Digestive Health:

- Surgical stress increases intestinal permeability[51]

- Surgical stress reduces blood supply (ischemia) to the colon[47]

- Surgical stress causes gastric ulcers[52]

- Surgical stress causes gastric bleeding[53]

Exercise:

- Surgical stress causes loss of muscle mass and strength[54]

Eye Health:

- Surgical stress causes vision loss[55]

Hair Health:

- Surgical stress causes hair loss (alopecia)[56]

Healing:

- Surgical stress impairs wound healing[57]

Hearing:

- Surgical stress causes hearing loss[58]

Heart Health:

- Surgical stress causes heart attack[59,60]

- Surgical stress causes heart failure[61,62]

Immune System:

- Surgical stress impairs the immune system[63]

- Surgical stress suppresses anti-tumor immunity[64]

- Surgical stress increases risk of infection[65]

Kidney Health:

- Surgical stress causes kidney dysfunction[47]

Liver Health:

- Surgical stress causes liver dysfunction[66]

- Surgical stress causes multiple organ failure[53]

Lung Health:

- Surgical stress causes collapsed lung (atelectasis)[67]

Sexual Health:

- Surgical stress causes erectile dysfunction[68]

- Surgical stress significantly decreases blood testosterone levels[69]

Sleep:

- Surgical stress reduces sleep quality[70]

Thyroid Health:

- Surgical stress lowers thyroid function[71]

Tumor Microenvironment:

The area surrounding a tumor, commonly referred to as the tumor microenvironment, is one of the most important areas of cancer research. Its significance stems from the fact that substances present within it are in constant interaction with cancer cells and can determine the fate of a tumor.

Listed below are many of the changes that occur within the tumor microenvironment as a result of surgery.

- Surgical stress increases free radicals[89]

- Surgical stress increases high mobility group box 1 protein[73]

- Surgical stress increases tumor necrosis factor-alpha[75]

- Surgical stress increases interleukin-1beta[77]

- Surgical stress increases interleukin-4[74]

- Surgical stress increases interleukin-6[75,76]

- Surgical stress increases interleukin-8[75]

- Surgical stress increases nuclear factor-kappa b[72]

- Surgical stress increases cortisol[78]

- Surgical stress increases adrenaline[122]

- Surgical stress increases prolactin[35]

- Surgical stress increases vascular endothelial growth factor[79]

- Surgical stress increases epidermal growth factor[80]

- Surgical stress increases nitric oxide[82]

- Surgical stress increases lactic acid[100]

- Surgical stress increases estrogen[101]

- Surgical stress increases prostaglandins[102]

- Surgical stress increases serotonin[103]

- Surgical stress increases histamine[103]

16 WAYS SURGERY CAUSES CANCER

By investigating each individual factor found within the tumor microenvironment, we can pinpoint many of the ways cancer surgery promotes the growth and spread of cancer.

1. Nitric Oxide - Anytime a tissue has been injured, nitric oxide and other growth factors are released to signal cells to grow and divide to replace lost cells.[83] In a person with cancer, tumor cells caught in the crossfire of nitric oxide signaling will also be signaled to grow, which is why nitric oxide is a well-known promoter of angiogenesis and tumor progression.[84-87]

2. Nitric Oxide - Nitric oxide has also been demonstrated to trigger the adhesion of circulating tumor cells (like the ones released during cancer surgery) onto body tissues, which is the first step in new tumor formation.[88]

3. Vascular Endothelial Growth Factor – Similar to nitric oxide, VEGF is a protein that signals growth to help repair injured tissues.[124] Elevated blood levels of VEGF have been associated with the growth and progression of cancer.[125]

4. Epidermal Growth Factor – EGF, like nitric oxide and VEGF, enhances the growth, invasion and metastasis of tumors.[126] High levels of EGF are associated with poor prognosis in cancer patients.[127]

5. Free Radicals – Free radicals are highly-reactive molecules that are balanced by the body's antioxidant system. In excess, the oxidative damage caused by free radicals results in aging, cardiovascular disease, cancer and other chronic diseases.[148]

6. Adrenaline – The stress hormone adrenaline is one of the primary triggers of the breakdown of fat for energy (lipolysis).[123] Anytime unsaturated fatty acids enter the bloodstream, prostaglandins are formed,[90] which are carcinogenic.[91]

7. Cortisol - People with cancer have higher cortisol levels than people without cancer,[92] and a number of studies have shown that cancer patients with the highest levels of cortisol have the greatest risk of dying from the disease.[93,94]

8. Estrogen - The presence of cortisol in the bloodstream leads to increased production of the hormone estrogen.[95-97] The famous 1990's Women's Health Initiative study tested the effects of supplemental estrogen on women, but was forced to stop early after participants began developing cardiovascular disease, stroke, dementia and cancer.[98]

9. Serotonin - Since cortisol's basic action is to catabolize muscle tissue and muscle meat contains high levels of the amino acid tryptophan (a precursor for serotonin), stress increases serotonin production.[104] While most people think of serotonin as a 'happy hormone,' this cultural belief appears misguided, since serotonin is not a hormone and lowering it can alleviate depression.[120] Serotonin is part of the body's stress response and has been shown in numerous studies to promote tumor growth.[104-108]

10. Histamine - Histamine is an inflammatory mediator commonly known for its role in allergic reactions.[109,110] Substances that inhibit histamine prevent cancer growth and progression.[111-113]

11. Lactic Acid - Lactic acid is produced by cells that aren't getting what they need to produce energy efficiently. Lactic acid suppresses the immune system,[114] promotes cancer growth and metastasis[115] and also triggers the release of cortisol,[116] perpetuating the cycle of stress.

12. Prolactin - Elevated blood concentrations of the hormone prolactin trigger inflammation by amplifying the production of inflammatory cytokines,[117] and promote the formation and progression of numerous types of cancer. [118,119,121]

13. Tumor Necrosis Factor alpha – TNFalpha is an inflammatory cytokine released by macrophages in response to toxins or other stressors.[129] Due to its extreme toxicity, TNFalpha has been shown to kill cancer cells,[130] but the rest of the body is severely damaged in the process.[131-133] TNFalpha promotes inflammation, is involved in cancer growth and metastasis, and its presence in the body increases with age,[134] like cancer's.[135]

14. Nuclear Factor Kappa b – TNFalpha triggers the production of NFKB,[136] which is a protein that signals inflammation[137] and plays a key role in tumor formation, growth and spread.[138,139] Many ancient natural medicines found to be effective against cancer inhibit NFKB.[140]

15. Interleukin 6 – IL-6 is a highly-toxic pro-inflammatory cytokine[141,142] that plays a key role in the formation of numerous types of cancer, including colorectal,[128] pancreatic,[146] liver[147] and prostate.[81]

16. High-Mobility Group Box 1 Protein – HMGB1 is a pro-inflammatory protein that signals immune system activation in response to injury.[149] Overexpression of HMGB1 promotes inflammation, carcinogenesis, angiogenesis and metastasis. "Our studies and those of our colleagues suggest that HMGB1 is central to cancer."[145]

In conclusion, surgical removal of a tumor triggers the release of an assortment of substances that each play important roles in cancer growth, progression and metastasis. However, it isn't just cancer surgery that promotes the growth and spread of cancer: *All forms of surgery* promote the growth and spread of cancer - even in people who don't have cancer.[99]

TIMELESS QUOTES

"Modern cancer surgery someday will be regarded with the same kind of horror that we now regard the use of leeches in George Washington's time."
- Dr. Robert Mendelsohn

"The disease always returns after removal, and operation only accelerates its growth and fatal termination."
- Alfred-Armand-Louis-Marie Velpeau, Surgeon (1795-1867)

"I do not despair of carcinoma being cured somewhere in the future, but this blessed achievement will, I believe, never be wrought by the knife of the surgeon."
- Dr. Hayes Agnew (1818-1892)

CHAPTER 2

CHEMOTHERAPY

CHEMOTHERAPY IS A cancer treatment in which highly-toxic chemicals are injected into patients in an attempt to kill cancer cells. The first chemotherapeutic agent ever used, which is still being administered to this day, is a derivative of the chemical weapon mustard gas, called mustargen.

The United States learned a lot about mustard gas during World War II, where damaged bone marrow and lymph tissues seen in autopsies of exposed soldiers revealed the weapon's prime target: the immune system.[1] Even more was learned about the effects of mustard gas when the US government conducted a series of secret tests on 60,000 of its own troops. *National Public Radio* broke the story in 2015,

---

"Sixty-thousand American troops served as test subjects, and about 4,000 were used in extreme tests that government studies have linked to illnesses including skin cancer, leukemia and chronic breathing problems. The test subjects were sworn to secrecy until the program was formally declassified in 1993. By then, the youngest World War II veterans were in their 60s and 70s. Many of the men in the experiments never shared the details with their families."[2]

FROM BATTLEFIELD TO CANCER CLINIC

What do you do after discovering a chemical weapon that knocks out the immune system, causes cancer and makes exposed skin literally slough off the body? Naturally you dispose of it – as safely as possible – and stop its production forever. But while mustard gas has been banned on the battlefield by international treaties,[3] instead of leaving this devastating poison behind us as a dark remnant of our past to be revisited only in history books – the government decided to begin injecting it into sick people with cancer.

After World War II ended, the US Department of Defense funded Dr. Goodman and Dr. Gilman of Yale University to administer mustard gas to rats and observe its effects on tumors. Their tumors regressed. They tested it on a lymphoma patient with advanced cancer and their tumors also regressed.[4-6] So amazed was the medical community that a drug could cause tumor regression, that it didn't seem to matter the patient died within a couple of months.

Interestingly, around this same time Dr. Gerson – an American physician famous for his nutritional approach to cancer, which included fresh fruit and vegetable juices, liver extract injections, thyroid hormone, coffee enemas and other nutrients – presented cases to US congress of cancer patients he had allegedly cured using his nutritional therapy.[7] The world of medicine was at a fork in the road, Dr. Nicholas Gonzales explains, "it could have gone toward natural treatments, it could have gone toward synthetic. But because of that extraordinary response in a single patient that lasted a few weeks, the entire chemo industry came into fruition."[8]

WARNING LABEL FOR MUSTARGEN

"This drug is HIGHLY TOXIC and both powder and solution must be handled and administered with care. Inhalation of dust or vapors and contact with skin or mucous membranes, especially those of the eyes, must be avoided. Avoid exposure during pregnancy. Due to the toxic properties of mechlorethamine (e.g., corrosivity, carcinogenicity, mutagenicity, teratogenicity), special handling procedures should be reviewed prior to handling and followed diligently. Extravasation of the drug into subcutaneous tissues results in a painful inflammation. The area usually becomes indurated and sloughing may occur."[18]

CHEMOTHERAPY VS. CANCER

It doesn't take more than common sense to reason that injecting poison into the veins of a sick person will 1) not cure them and 2) probably make their health worse. A study published in *The Lancet* in 1980 found that of 78 patients who received chemotherapy, survival "was no better than that of the 80 who did not receive chemotherapy." Furthermore, regression of tumors was found to have no impact on survival and, "survival may even have been shortened in some patients given chemotherapy," the study reports.[9]

The most comprehensive review ever conducted on the efficacy of chemotherapy was completed by German epidemiologist and biostatistician Dr. Ulrich Abel. Europe's most popular news magazine *Der Spiegel*, which sells over 1-million copies per week, featured Dr. Abel's publication in a 2004 article titled *Useless Poisonous Cures (Giftkur ohne Nutzen)*.[10] In order to obtain every study and clinical trial ever published on chemotherapy, Dr. Abel sent letters to over 350 medical centers across the world; his review consisted of thousands of studies and took two years to complete.

Dr. Abel pronounced that despite new and increasingly expensive poisons being used during chemotherapy, "patients do not live a day longer" than they did 25 years prior. Overall worldwide chemotherapy success rates he said were "appalling," and that "for most internal cancers no proof exists that chemotherapy, especially the increasingly high dose variety, increases life expectancy or improves quality of life." Dr. Abel estimated at least 80% of chemotherapy administered throughout the world is completely worthless.[11]

A group of Australian scientists published a study in 2004 suggesting that *far more* than just 80% of chemotherapy administered is worthless. During a follow-up with cancer patients 5-years after receiving chemotherapy, the researchers determined that only 2.1% of patients in the US and 2.3% of patients in Australia were still alive – exposing chemotherapy's astonishing 98% failure rate.[12] *I wonder how many of these patients would have been alive at 5-years if they hadn't received chemotherapy.*

Seeking a greater understanding of what happens inside the body after an injection of chemotherapy, scientists from Harvard Medical School and the University of Massachusetts tested 88 currently-used chemotherapeutic drugs on fruit flies in 2013. Michelle Markstein, molecular biologist and co-author of the study reported, "...several chemotherapeutics that stop fast growing tumors have the opposite effect on stem cells in the same animal, causing them to divide too rapidly."[13] By shrinking the initial tumor mass, chemotherapy deceives doctors into thinking patients are benefitting from the treatment, when in actuality, the growth and spread of cancer are being accelerated by it.

Another way of analyzing the effects of chemotherapy on human health is to look at people who were involved in producing it during times of war. Retired Japanese poison gas factory workers were evaluated 57-years after they had been manufacturing mustard gas during World

War II. The study found that exposure to mustard gas "significantly increases the long-term risk of death from respiratory cancer and chronic bronchitis/emphysema."[84]

For the first time ever, researchers investigated chemotherapy-induced death at a number of hospitals in the UK. Published in the esteemed journal *Lancet Oncology* in 2016, the study found that 8.4% of people undergoing chemotherapy for lung cancer and 2.4% of people treated for breast cancer nationwide were killed by the treatment within 30-days of administration. When they looked at the numbers from the Milton Keynes Hospital they discovered an even more startling figure: 50.9% of lung cancer patients were killed by chemotherapy within 30-days of treatment.[14]

SUCCESS STORIES?

One Cancer Patient's Experience with Chemotherapy

"This highly toxic fluid was being injected into my veins. The nurse administering it was wearing protective gloves because it would burn her skin if just a tiny drip came into contact with it. I couldn't help asking myself 'If such precautions are needed to be taken on the outside, what is it doing to me on the inside?' From 7 pm that evening, I vomited solidly for two and a half days. During my treatment, I lost my hair by the handful, I lost my appetite, my skin colour, my zest for life. I was death on legs," described a cancer patient in the book *Now and Then* by Bob Madison.

Women Struggling to Live Normal Lives Following Chemotherapy

Thousands of women who have received chemotherapy for breast cancer are struggling to live normal lives, reports a 2016 study published in the journal *Cancer*.

Just one year after treatment, 20% of women above the age of 65 were so debilitated that they couldn't carry out basic daily tasks like walking across the room, light housework, shopping, kneeling or standing long enough to shower.[15]

Cancer Patient Survives Decades Until Chemotherapy

The longest-surviving breast cancer patient of all-time was diagnosed at age 45 and lived until she was 93-years-old. Following her diagnosis, she received no treatment for 22 years, at which point doctors discovered metastatic cancer in her lungs and put her on estrogen-inhibiting drugs.

14 years later, they found cancer on her spine and put her on a different estrogen inhibitor. Years later, doctors found cancer in her liver and finally decided to try chemotherapy.

After receiving two cycles of the chemotherapy drug capecitabine, she refused further treatment due to intolerable side effects, and was dead within two years.[16]

ADDITIONAL HEALTH EFFECTS

Despite careful adherence to a strict set of safety protocols for handling chemotherapy drugs, including the use of personal protective equipment, more than half of nursing and pharmacy workers in a 2016 study reported complaints of dizziness simply from working with chemotherapy drugs.[17]

Side effects of chemotherapy include, but are not limited to:

Blood Health:

- Chemotherapy decreases red blood cells (anemia)[19]

- Chemotherapy decreases white blood cells (leukopenia)[20]

- Chemotherapy decreases blood platelets (thrombocytopenia)[21]

Bone Health:

- Chemotherapy causes bone death (osteonecrosis)[22]

- Chemotherapy causes loss of bone mineral density (osteoporosis)[23,24]

Brain Health:

- Chemotherapy is toxic to the brain (neurotoxic)[25]

- Chemotherapy causes long-lasting impairment of concentration, forgetfulness and slower thinking; termed "chemobrain" [26,27]

- Chemotherapy causes altered consciousness[28]

- Chemotherapy causes degeneration of white matter in the brain (leukoencephalopathy) [28]

- Chemotherapy causes nerve damage (neuropathy) [28]

- Chemotherapy causes seizures[28]

- Chemotherapy causes paralysis[28]

- Chemotherapy causes stroke (cerebral infarction) [28]

Digestive Health:

- Chemotherapy causes diarrhea[36]

- Chemotherapy causes painful inflammation and ulceration in the digestive tract (intestinal mucositis)[41]

- Chemotherapy causes "significant intestinal damage in both jejunum and colon"[37]

Exercise:

- Chemotherapy reduces grip strength[38]

- Chemotherapy causes muscle dysfunction and a loss of overall strength[39]

Eye Health:

- Chemotherapy causes severe vision loss and altered color vision[40]

- Chemotherapy causes complete blindness[41]

Hair Health:

- Chemotherapy causes hair loss[50]

Healing:

- Chemotherapy impairs wound healing[51]

Hearing:

- Chemotherapy causes "severe to profound hearing loss"[52]

- Chemotherapy causes chronic ringing of the ears (tinnitus)[52]

Heart Health:

- Chemotherapy damages the heart[53]

- Chemotherapy causes heart disease[54]

- Chemotherapy causes heart failure[55]

- Chemotherapy causes heart attacks (myocardial infarction)[56]

Immune System:

- Chemotherapy causes long-term immune system damage[57,58]

- Chemotherapy exacerbates existing hepatitis C infections[59]

- Chemotherapy reactivates hepatitis B virus[60]

- Chemotherapy impairs anti-tumor immune response[61]

Kidney Health:

- Chemotherapy causes kidney failure[65]

Liver Health:

- Chemotherapy causes liver injury[66]

Lung Health:

- Chemotherapy causes lung disease[67]

Mental Health:

- Chemotherapy "decreased emotional and social function and increased distress"[29]

- Chemotherapy causes depression[30]

- Chemotherapy causes anxiety[31]

Oral Health:

- Chemotherapy causes severe dental caries[32]

- Chemotherapy causes dry mouth (xerostomia), ulcers and mouth sores[68]

- Chemotherapy causes oral candida (fungal) infection[33]

- Chemotherapy causes painful inflammation and ulceration in the mouth (oral mucositis)[34]

- Chemotherapy causes "a diverse spectrum of oral changes that generally are attributed to immunosuppression and bleeding tendencies"[35]

Pain:

- Chemotherapy causes neuropathic pain; burning or coldness, "pins and needles" sensations, numbness and itching[69]

- Chemotherapy pain remains one-year after treatment[70]

Quality of Life:

- Chemotherapy causes difficulty swallowing (dysphagia)[71]

- Chemotherapy causes nausea and vomiting (emesis)[72,73]

- Chemotherapy causes altered taste sensation[74]

- Chemotherapy causes migraine headaches[75]

Sexual Health:

- Chemotherapy causes infertility and premature ovarian failure;[42,43] in up to 66% of women[44]

- Chemotherapy causes absence of menstrual period (amenorrhea)[45]

- Chemotherapy causes menopausal symptoms[45]

- Chemotherapy damages sperm and testicular tissue"[46,47]

- Chemotherapy reduces reproductive organ weight, sperm count and sperm motility[46]

- Chemotherapy causes "a significant decline in serum testosterone"[46]

- Chemotherapy causes erectile dysfunction[48,49]

Skin:

- Chemotherapy causes dermatitis: itchiness, red skin, or a rash[76]

Sleep:

- Chemotherapy reduces sleep quality[77]

Thyroid Health:

- Chemotherapy "blunts thyroid function"[78]

- Chemotherapy impairs thyroid hormone synthesis and secretion from the thyroid gland[79]

- Thyroid hormones "...were remarkably altered after each cycle of chemotherapy leading to decline in thyroid function..."[80]

Tumor Microenvironment:

- Chemotherapy increases free radicals[85]

- Chemotherapy increases cortisol[85]

- Chemotherapy increases adrenaline[93]

- Chemotherapy increases prolactin[94]

- Chemotherapy increases estrogen[64]

- Chemotherapy increases tumor necrosis factor-alpha[62]

- Chemotherapy increases interleukin 1- beta[62]

- Chemotherapy increases interleukin-6[91]

- Chemotherapy increases interleukin-8[92]

- Chemotherapy increases nuclear factor-kappa b[62]

- Chemotherapy increases prostaglandins[86]

- Chemotherapy increases nitric oxide[46]

- Chemotherapy increases vascular endothelial growth factor[95]

- Chemotherapy increases epidermal growth factor[96]

- Chemotherapy increases lactic acid[87]

- Chemotherapy increases serotonin[88]

- Chemotherapy increases histamine[89]

- Chemotherapy increases high-mobility group box 1 protein[90]

Urinary Health:

- Chemotherapy causes blood in the urine (hematuria)[81]

- Chemotherapy causes painful urination (dysuria)[81]

Weight Loss:

- Chemotherapy causes muscle-wasting (cachexia)[82]

- "Severe loss of body weight (cachexia) is a frequent cause of death in cancer patients and is exacerbated by chemotherapy"[83]

TIMELESS QUOTES

"Most cancer patients in this country die of chemotherapy. Chemotherapy does not eliminate breast, colon, or lung cancers. This fact has been documented for over a decade, yet doctors still use chemotherapy for these tumors."
- Dr. Allen Levin, The Healing of Cancer

"As a chemist trained to interpret data, it is incomprehensible to me that physicians can ignore the clear evidence that chemotherapy does much, much more harm than good."
- Alan Nixon, Ph.D., Past President of The American Chemical Society

"Chemotherapy and radiotherapy will make the ancient method of drilling holes in a patient's head to permit the escape of demons look relatively advanced. Toxic chemotherapy is a hoax. The doctors who use it are guilty of pre-meditated murder, and the use of cobalt and other methods of cancer treatment popular today effectively closes the door on cure."
- Ernst T. Krebs Jr., American Biochemist (1911-1996)

"To sell chemotherapy as a 'therapy' is most likely the biggest deceit in the history of medicine. Whoever masterminded this chemo-torture deserves a monument in hell."
- Dr. Ryke Geerd Hamer, M.D.

CHAPTER 3

RADIOTHERAPY

RADIOTHERAPY, ALSO KNOWN as radiation therapy, is a treatment in which ionizing x-ray and gamma ray radiation are directed at tumors and used to kill cancer cells. Blasting cells with radiation stops them from growing and multiplying, but it also damages every other cell in its path and sets in motion a cascade of negative physiological effects that can persist for multiple generations.

Today, up to 60% of cancer patients receive radiotherapy as a part of their treatment regimens[1] and yet most are never fully aware of the risks involved with exposure to ionizing radiation.

THE DISCOVERY OF X-RAYS

X-rays were first discovered in 1895 by German physics professor Wilhelm Röntgen. In 1901, Röntgen was awarded the Nobel Prize for his discovery and ironically, both he and his wife ended up dying from cancer caused by x-ray exposure.[2]

With the advent of a machine that could produce x-rays, suddenly the medical industry had an impressive new way to destroy cells other than cauterizing or burning with acid; and within a few years, ionizing radiation was put to use on cancer patients. However, a number of common side effects quickly became known, including burns, skin disease and the formation of tumors, but society failed to take these warnings seriously and by 1922, over 100 radiologists and many others working in the medical industry had died from cancer caused by x-rays.[3] And yet the ignorance continued...

SHOE-FITTING X-RAY FLUOROSCOPES

In the 1920's, portable x-ray devices became widely available in shoe stores so customers could see the bones in their feet to determine which shoes were the right fit - and kids loved them![4] At the peak of popularity in the United States, there were at least 10,000 shoe-fitting x-ray fluoroscopes in use, and despite the massive radiation exposure (equal to more than 1000 chest x-rays) and the significant amount of scatter radiation emitted from these "cancer boxes," the horrifying nature of the technology was largely brushed off by the government and medical community.

By the 1970's, the incidence of foot cancer spiked dramatically and the negative effects could no longer be denied.[5] The shoe-fitting fluoroscopes used in shoe stores for around 50-years had officially been banned.

FLUOROSCOPES AS ENTERTAINMENT

After World War II, every physician in America was urged to have an x-ray fluoroscope in their office and no examination was considered complete unless patients were fluoroscoped.[6] In the 1940's, some pediatricians used fluoroscopes on babies every single month during checkups for the first two years of life.[6] Doctors would flaunt their fancy fluoroscopes to patients as a source of entertainment, which Dr. Raymond Peat, endocrinologist, physiologist and science historian described as "a combination of ignorance and arrogance."[7] It seems society was obsessed with technology in much the same way we are today with computers, cell phones and other gadgets.

RADIOTHERAPY VS. CANCER

During the Chernobyl nuclear disaster in 1986, massive amounts of radioactive isotopes billowed up into the atmosphere before reigning down onto most of Europe – and nobody exposed to fallout from this catastrophe was cured of cancer. In fact, the largest and most comprehensive mortality study on the Chernobyl disaster to date, which included data from over 1000 published studies and over 5000 internet and printed publications, concluded that between the years 1986 and 2004, the radioactivity released by this event caused 985,000 deaths, mostly from cancer.[8]

RADIOTHERAPY ADMINISTERS 5X THE FATAL DOSE

Emeritus Professor of Physics at the University of Oxford Wade Allison briefly discussed radiotherapy in a 2012 report on Nuclear Technology.[9]   Over the course of a month, he wrote, "the tumour gets more than 40,000 mSv [millisieverts] and the peripheral healthy tissue as much as 20,000 mSv – that is five times the fatal dose experienced by some Chernobyl workers." In other words, if radiotherapy doses weren't spread out over the course of a month or longer, every patient receiving it would die instantly.

RADIOTHERAPY FOR BREAST CANCER

Since radiotherapy first came onto the scene, the standard of care for women with breast cancer was surgical breast removal (radical mastectomy) followed by radiotherapy. However, at the time this regimen was put into practice, scientific research hadn't even established that it was beneficial for patients; and up until 1960, a large amount of conflicting research had been published:

- Some studies indicated radiotherapy following radical mastectomy provided good results[10-14]

- Others reported no benefit from the treatment[15-23]

- And several suggested radiotherapy was harmful[24,25]

The National Cancer Institute responded to this uncertainty in 1961 by launching *The National Surgical Adjuvant Breast and Bowel Project* (NSABP). For the project, American scientist Bernard Fisher and his colleagues compared the efficacy of mastectomy alone with mastectomy followed by irradiation. Published in the *Annals of Surgery* in 1970, the study found that radiotherapy *decreased survival of all patients*. "Survival of patients was determined 3, 4 and 5 years following operation…At each time, survival of those irradiated was slightly less than in the control patients."[26]

In 1974, researchers from the Swiss Institute for Experimental Cancer Research examined survival rates of women from six clinical trials who received either radical mastectomy or radical mastectomy followed by irradiation for breast cancer. Published in *The Lancet*, scientists concluded, "An increased mortality in early breast cancer can be correlated to the routine use of local postoperative irradiation. The decreased survival is statistically significant. Of controlled clinical trials so far published, all six, including more than 3400 patients, demonstrate decreased survival of between 1 and 10% in irradiated patients when compared with those treated by mastectomy alone."[27]

In 1995, a meta-analysis of 64 randomized trials was conducted to find out if irradiation following either mastectomy or lumpectomy improves survival of patients with breast cancer. Published in *The New England Journal of Medicine*, the study reports, "The addition of radiotherapy to surgery resulted in...no significant difference in 10-year survival."[28]

So far the evidence suggests that at best, radiotherapy doesn't improve survival of breast cancer patients, and at worst, radiotherapy is killing cancer patients more quickly than they would have died without it. Couple these findings with similar findings about radiotherapy following lung cancer surgery and it seems likely that the latter is true.

RADIOTHERAPY FOR LUNG CANCER

A 1998 review of nine randomized trials compared survival rates of 2,128 lung cancer patients who received radiotherapy following surgery with patients who received surgery alone. Published in *The Lancet*, results showed that patients who received radiotherapy following surgery had a 27% increased risk of death. Researchers concluded that, "Postoperative radiotherapy is detrimental to patients with early-stage completely resected NSCLC [non-small-cell lung cancer] and should not be used routinely for such patients."[29]

Scientists from the United Kingdom conducted an extensive review in 2005 evaluating the efficacy of radiotherapy following surgery in patients with non-small-cell lung cancer. Published in the journal *Lung Cancer,* they wrote, "Results continue to show PORT [postoperative radiotherapy] to be detrimental, with an 18% relative increase in the risk of death."[30]

WHISTLEBLOWER EXPOSES CANCER MORTALITY STATISTICS

One of the most fascinating statements made by whistleblower Dr. Ralph Moss in his book *The Cancer Industry* is that official cancer mortality statistics are being intentionally manipulated in order to make it appear like cancer treatments are better than they actually are.

Since radiotherapy damages all organs and systems of the body, including the brain,[96-99] heart,[110-115] liver,[128-129] kidneys,[127] thyroid,[157] immune system,[116-125] and impairs the healing process,[103-105] there are endless ways that its side effects can eventually kill a person. One of the most common ways is heart disease;[110-115] so what Dr. Moss was referring to, was the fact that if a patient receives radiotherapy then has a heart attack and dies a week, month or even a few years later, their cause of death will be deemed a heart attack rather than a cancer death due to treatment failure; and consequently, the public never finds out just how unsuccessful radiotherapy actually is. Evidence of this can be seen in studies reporting decreased cancer deaths while simultaneously reporting increased non-cancer deaths following radiotherapy treatment.[28,32,33]

In 1993, Texas researchers from the Anderson Cancer Center in Houston questioned the validity of official government cancer mortality statistics by examining non-cancer deaths of 470,000 cancer patients. Published in the *Journal of the National Cancer Institute*, the study found that 27% of patients who were reported dead for reasons other than cancer had died within a year after diagnosis, suggesting they were probably killed by their treatments; "…it appears that this excess was caused by treatment of the cancer." [31] In other words, cancer treatments are less effective than we're told and the true death toll from cancer is actually much greater than we're told.

RADIOTHERAPY ELEVATES LIFETIME RISK OF CANCER

Whether radiotherapy treatment is used for acne, peptic ulcers, scalp ringworm or cancer, universally we see an elevated risk of cancer that lasts for the remainder of the patient's life.[34] For example, a 36-year-old male patient who was treated with radiotherapy and chemotherapy for Hodgkin's disease in 1972 developed colon cancer 18 years later.[35]

"Indeed, young patients treated with chemotherapy and especially radiation therapy are at high risk of developing secondary cancers. Chemo-radiotherapy appears to also increase more significantly the risk."[36] What's more, the risk of secondary cancers developing later in life is even greater for those treated during childhood; "Risks of radiation-related cancer are greatest for those exposed early in life, and these risks appear to persist throughout life."[37]

- Radiotherapy for scalp ringworm causes multiple basal cell carcinomas in about 40% of patients up to 50 years later.[38]

- Radiotherapy for acne is strongly associated with basal cell carcinoma arising within the radiation treatment field.[39]

- Radiotherapy for Hodgkin's lymphoma in children increases breast cancer risk 24-times.[40]

- Radiotherapy for Hodgkin's lymphoma increases stomach cancer risk 3.4-times[41]

- Radiotherapy for Hodgkin's lymphoma increases the risk of breast cancer, "…with risk increasing dramatically more than 15 years after therapy."[42]

- Radiotherapy for testicular cancer increases pancreatic cancer risk 2.9-times, persisting for over 20 years.[43]

- Radiotherapy for testicular cancer increases stomach cancer risk 5.9-times, persisting "for several decades."[44]

- Radiotherapy for breast cancer significantly increases cancer formation in the other (contralateral) breast[33]

- Radiotherapy for peptic ulcers increases risk of cancer; "Cancer mortality remained high for up to 50 years, indicating that radiation damage may persist to the end of life."[45]

What is happening inside the body as a result of exposure to ionizing radiation that causes lifelong damage?

RADIATION BYSTANDER EFFECTS

To this day, mainstream theory states that radiation kills cancer cells by directly damaging DNA.[46] However, in 1992, Harvard researchers discovered something that called the entire theory into question:[47] when a cell is irradiated, something is emitted by the injured cell that transfers the same damage to non-irradiated cells – a term called a 'bystander effect.'[48]

A colorful demonstration of bystander effects was performed by researchers at McMaster University in Ontario, Canada in 2006, where scientist Carmel E. Mothersill and her colleagues irradiated rainbow trout (0.5 Gy dose) and then placed them in water-filled containers with non-irradiated fish. Two days later, they discovered that the damage had been transferred from the irradiated fish to the non-irradiated fish – an effect that was said to be caused by the "secretion of a chemical messenger into the water."[49]

Bystander effects have also been demonstrated in animals,[50,51,52] in humans,[53,54] and even in plants.[55]

A CLOSER LOOK...

Chinese researchers irradiated the roots of young Arabidopsis thaliana plants to determine if it would cause bystander effects. As the plant grew, researchers found evidence of radiation damage "in every true leaf over the course of rosette development." They even found damage in non-irradiated plants that were nearby.[55]

In 2008, researchers from Alberta, Canada irradiated the heads of mice "while the remainder of the body was completely protected by a medical-grade shield." They discovered DNA damage, altered cellular growth and cell death in shielded spleen cells.[52]

Scientists from the University of Washington investigated the effects of dental x-rays on pregnant women and their offspring in 2004. Even though the women were entirely shielded with lead aprons during the X-ray images, irradiation damage was transferred to the fetus and many of the babies were born underweight.[54]

What is the chemical messenger released by irradiated cells that causes bystander effects?

Although at least one other factor is involved,[56] by far the major facilitator of bystander effects is nitric oxide (NO). Nitric oxide's effects include genomic instability,[57] genetic errors,[57] double-strand DNA breaks,[58] cell death (apoptosis),[59] inflammation,[59] and ultimately, carcinogenesis.[78,79] Lowering nitric oxide levels (for example, by supplementing with an inexpensive, medicinal blue dye called methylene blue[60]) can 'switch off' bystander effects and halt the self-perpetuating cycle of damage.[61]

Interestingly, the effects of ionizing radiation appear to be indistinguishable from estrogen,[62] and since estrogen rapidly elevates levels of nitric oxide in the body,[63,64] lowering estrogen is probably a more fundamental way to interrupt bystander effects.

When any part of the body is exposed to ionizing radiation, even at the low-doses commonly used during medical x-rays,[65] nitric oxide-mediated bystander effects transfer the damage to unexposed body parts - but it goes beyond that.

In 2010, researchers from Texas discovered that millimeter waves - a much less intense form of radiation that's often used at airport security checkpoints - can also induce bystander effects.[66]

Biochemist Martin Pall of Washington State University tested even lower frequencies to see if they could induce bystander effects in 2013. Published in the journal *Bioelectromagnetics*, Pall found that microwave and even extra-low frequency (ELF) radiation - the kind emitted from cell phones and other wireless devices - both induce nitric oxide synthesis.[67] This suggests that both non-ionizing microwave and ELF radiation will have some of the same effects as ionizing radiation. And indeed, there is abundant evidence within the scientific literature associating cell phone use with cancer; including brain tumors[68-73] mouth cancer,[74] lymphoma,[75] breast cancer[76] and eye cancer.[77]

SUCCESS STORIES?

Richard Wayman

One year after 59-year-old Richard Wayman received radiotherapy for cancer of the tonsils, he began feeling a "painful tingling" in his legs. Within weeks, he was struggling to walk and was admitted to the hospital for x-rays, scans and other tests.

"The scans revealed lesions on my lungs, which raised fears that the cancer had spread, so I was admitted to another hospital for a biopsy and, as a result, contracted MRSA [infection] and pneumonia."

During his time spent in the hospital to treat his conditions, Richard lost around 50 lbs. "I thought I was never going to get out of there," he remarked. Finally, doctors diagnosed his lung lesions as a side-effect of radiotherapy, but his problems continued.

After having a tooth pulled by his dentist, the bone around the extracted tooth "started to crumble and become infected."

Within a couple months he had an open wound running from his outer cheek through his jaw bone and into his mouth, called bone necrosis - another side effect of radiotherapy.[91]

Scott Jerome-Parks and Alexandra Jn-Charles

Anytime technology is involved there is the potential that it could malfunction. Although rare, errors during radiotherapy administration have occurred and the results have been disastrous.

Cancer patient Scott Jerome-Parks was overdosed with radiation that left him burnt, deaf, visually impaired, with ulcers in his mouth, teeth falling out, unable to swallow or breathe and dead several painful weeks later.

Another victim of technological failure was 32-year-old breast cancer patient Alexandra Jn-Charles, who received 27 days of radiation overdoses that burnt a hole in her chest and left a gaping wound so painful that it made her consider suicide. [93]

ADDITIONAL HEALTH EFFECTS

Here's a list of side effects of radiotherapy reported in the scientific literature.

Bone Health:

- Radiotherapy damages the spinal cord[93]

- Radiotherapy causes bone fractures[94]

- Radiotherapy causes bone and joint degeneration[95]

Brain Health:

- Radiotherapy lowers IQ[96]

- Radiotherapy impairs memory, attention, and executive function[97,98]

- Radiotherapy increases lifetime risk of having a stroke[99]

Eye Health:

- Radiotherapy causes vision loss[100]

- Radiotherapy causes complete blindness[101]

Hair Health:

- Radiotherapy causes complete hair loss (alopecia)[102]

Healing:

- Radiotherapy slows wound healing[103-105]

Hearing:

- Radiotherapy causes immediate partial or total deafness[106] in 45.71% of patients[107]

- Radiotherapy-induced hearing loss continues to worsen over time[108,109]

Heart Health:

- Radiotherapy causes micro-vascular damage to the heart[112]

- Radiotherapy weakens the heart, blood vessels surrounding the heart and narrows arteries[113]

- Radiotherapy significantly increases mortality from cardiovascular death more than 15 years later[110-115]

Immune System:

- Radiotherapy suppresses the immune system[116]

- Radiotherapy inhibits anti-tumor immunity[116]

- Radiotherapy significantly increases risk of infection[117-124]

- "Immunity in young adult survivors of childhood leukemia [who received chemotherapy and/or radiotherapy] is similar to the elderly rather than age-matched controls"[125]

Inflammation:

- Radiotherapy causes immediate inflammation[126]

Kidney Health:

- Radiotherapy causes kidney failure[127]

Liver Health:

- Radiotherapy causes liver disease[128]

- Radiotherapy causes liver failure[129]

Mental Health:

- Radiotherapy causes mental disorders, anxiety, depression and distress[131,132]

- Radiotherapy causes "significantly worse mental health before, during and 1 year after RT [radiotherapy] compared to the normal population." [133]

Muscle-Loss:

- Radiation-induced cachexia causes primates to lose as much as 50% of skeletal muscle[134]

Oral Health:

- Radiotherapy causes tooth decay[135]

- Radiotherapy causes jaw bone death (osteoradionecrosis)[136]

- Radiotherapy causes permanent salivary gland dysfunction[137]

- Radiotherapy causes restricted mouth opening (trismus)[130]

- Radiotherapy causes oral discomfort, oral mucositis, changes in taste, increased oral infections and difficulty swallowing (dysphagia)[138]

Post-Traumatic Stress:

- Radiotherapy causes post-traumatic stress disorder[139]

Quality of Life:

- Radiotherapy causes fatigue in up to 90% of patients[140]

- Radiotherapy causes intractable (untreatable) nausea, vomiting and headache[141]

- Radiotherapy causes unpredictable taste and smell changes in 48% of patients; some had a stronger sweet taste, some had a stronger salt taste and some a weaker sense of smell[142]

- Radio-chemotherapy causes 64% of patients to rely on tube feeding as their primary means of food intake[143]

- Radiotherapy considerably impairs overall quality of life[144,145]

Sexual Health:

- Radiotherapy causes "…increased incidence of numerical sex chromosomal abnormalities and high risk for reproductive and genetic diseases…"[146]

- Total-body irradiation causes an "extremely high rate of gonadal dysfunction"[147]

- Radiotherapy causes a high percentage of infertility in cervical and testicular cancer patients[148]

- Radiotherapy causes sexual dysfunction in 78% of women treated for cervical cancer[149]

- Radiotherapy causes testosterone deficiency[150]

- Radiotherapy causes erectile dysfunction in 93.9% of men after prostate irradiation[151]

Skin:

- Radiotherapy causes thickening and scarring of skin and connective tissues[152]

- Shoe-fitting fluoroscopes cause dermatitis with ulceration on foot[153]

Sleep:

- Radiotherapy causes sleep problems in nearly half of patients[154]

- Radiotherapy causes severe obstructive sleep apnea[155]

Speech:

- Radiotherapy causes degeneration of voice and speech[156]

Thyroid Health:

- Radiotherapy causes hypothyroidism in approximately 53% of patients[157]

Tumor Microenvironment:

- Radiotherapy increases free radicals[164]

- Radiotherapy increases cortisol[80]

- Radiotherapy increases adrenaline[165]

- Radiotherapy increases estrogen[62]

- Radiotherapy increases prolactin[166]

- Radiotherapy increases nitric oxide[81]

- Radiotherapy increases vascular endothelial growth factor[82]

- Radiotherapy increases epidermal growth factor[83]

- Radiotherapy increases tumor necrosis factor alpha[88]

- Radiotherapy increases interleukin-1 beta[88]

- Radiotherapy increases interleukin-4[84]

- Radiotherapy increases interleukin-6[88]

- Radiotherapy increases interleukin-8[85]

- Radiotherapy increases nuclear factor kappa b[86]

- Radiotherapy increases prostaglandins[87]

- Radiotherapy increases lactic acid[167]

- Radiotherapy increases stem cell production[89,90]

- Radiotherapy increases histamine[161]

- Radiotherapy increases serotonin[162]

- Radiotherapy increases high-mobility group box 1 protein[163]

Urinary Health:

- Radiotherapy causes involuntary urination in women[158] and men[159]

- Radiotherapy for rectal cancer causes long-term incontinence and major disturbances in bowel function[160]

TIMELESS QUOTES

"… I wouldn't have chemotherapy and radiation because I'm not interested in therapies that cripple the immune system, and, in my opinion, virtually ensure failure for the majority of cancer patients."
- Dr Julian Whitaker, M.D.

"I had a brain cancer specialist sit in my living room and tell me that he would never take radiation if he had a brain tumor. And I asked him, 'but, do you send people for radiation?' and he said, of course. 'I'd be drummed out of the hospital if I didn't."
- Dr. Ralph Moss

CHAPTER 4

EARLY DETECTION, EARLY CURE?

LIKE ALL BUSINESSES, the cancer industry requires a steady flow of customers in order to generate revenue. The way it accomplishes this is by popularizing the idea that detecting and treating cancer in its early stages improves survival. 'Early detection saves lives' is a marketing strategy used to motivate people who have no signs or symptoms of cancer, to undergo regular screening for cancer.

The World Health Organization claims that "Cancer mortality can be reduced if cases are detected and treated early,"[1] and the American Cancer Society states, "Most doctors feel that early detection tests for breast cancer save thousands of lives each year. Many more lives probably could be saved if even more women and their health care providers took advantage of these tests."[2]

If early detection and treatment do in fact save lives, then this is indeed a righteous proposal, but the thing about 'early detection' is that - in order for it to be beneficial - the 'early treatment' that follows must be effective. And based on our investigations into orthodox cancer treatments in the preceding chapters, it seems incredibly unlikely that inflicting severe damage upon a sick person *at any stage* of their illness could improve their health. But rather than speculating, let's take a closer look at two of the most popular cancer screening tests and decide for ourselves if we think early detection saves lives.

THE PSA TEST: PROSTATE CANCER SCREENING

For a man, the road to being diagnosed with prostate cancer begins with a blood test called the prostate-specific antigen (PSA) test. A urologist might claim the PSA test is an accurate way to detect prostate cancer, but when we take a closer look, we come face-to-face with an uncomfortable reality: PSA cannot diagnose prostate cancer.[3] Dr. Richard Ablin - the man who discovered the prostate-specific antigen in 1970 - calls the widespread misuse of the PSA test "a public health disaster."

In his book *The Great Prostate Hoax*, Dr. Ablin reveals that prostate-specific antigen - a protein secreted by the prostate - is not cancer-specific. In other words, PSA is secreted by all prostates - both healthy and cancerous - and therefore, using it as a screening tool for prostate cancer is completely inappropriate.

If a man has his PSA levels tested and they end up being 4 or higher, the doctor will refer him to a urologist for a biopsy, which is the next step on the assembly line towards radiotherapy or surgical removal of the prostate (radical prostatectomy). But since PSA levels are increased by exercise, ejaculation and everyday stress, using them to determine whether or not a man is at risk for having cancer is no better than a coin toss. "You can biopsy according to whether a man has blue eyes or green eyes and get pretty much the same results as biopsying according to PSA," wrote Urologist Thomas Stamey, MD. "It is vital to understand that a man might have a PSA of 0.5 and have prostate cancer, yet another man whose number is an alarming 11 could be cancer free," Dr. Ablin explains.

Dr. Thomas Stamey and his colleagues at Stanford University studied prostate tissues collected over a 20-year period since the dawn of the PSA test in the early 1990's. Their 2004 study focused the scientific community's attention on what PSA-pioneer Dr. Richard Ablin had been saying for decades – the PSA test is virtually worthless in determining if men have prostate cancer; "the test indicates nothing more than the size of the prostate gland," Dr. Stamey declared, "The prostate specific antigen era in the united states is over."[4]

In 2011, the U.S. Preventive Services Task Force - an independent group of national experts in prevention and evidence-based medicine – reversed their previous position and recommended against the use of PSA screening with "moderate or high certainty that the service has no net benefit or that the harms outweigh the benefits."[5]

A CLOSER LOOK...

Scientists from Rockville, Maryland conducted an updated review on PSA screening in 2011. Results showed that "After about 10 years, PSA-based screening results in the detection of more cases of prostate cancer, but small to no reduction in prostate cancer-specific mortality."[6]

76,685 men aged 55-74 years were examined for prostate mortality after undergoing the PSA test in *The Prostate, Lung, Colorectal, and Ovarian (PLCO) Cancer Screening Trial* of 2012. Published in the *Journal of the National Cancer Institute*, the study found "no evidence of a mortality benefit for organized annual [PSA] screening" after 13-years of follow-up. In fact, prostate cancer mortality was slightly *increased* in the screened group: 3.7 per 10,000 person-years, versus 3.4 for unscreened men.[7]

A 2012 study published in *The New England Journal of Medicine* compared the efficacy of surgery versus no treatment in men diagnosed with prostate cancer by the PSA test. The study concluded that "radical prostatectomy [surgery] did not significantly reduce all-cause or prostate-cancer mortality, as compared with observation, through at least 12 years of follow-up."[8]

Despite clear evidence showing PSA screening fails to reduce mortality from prostate cancer[6-8] and the recommendation against the use of the PSA test by the Task Force, seductive celebrity-endorsed marketing campaigns pushing "prostate cancer awareness" continue luring men in to have their PSA's tested to this day.[9] Once the money train begins to roll, it can be difficult to stop.

"The prostate gland is at the epicenter of a worldwide trillion-dollar industry and the PSA test is its kingpin… if the test were made irrelevant, an industry would crumble."
- Dr. Richard Ablin

OVERDIAGNOSIS AND OVERTREATMENT

Of the 3.7 million men diagnosed with prostate cancer in the US between 1986 and 2005, "our paper estimates about 1.3 million are attributable solely to the test… and would not have occurred without it," said Dr. H. Gilbert Welch about his 2009 study published in the *Journal of the National Cancer Institute.*[10]

If the PSA test was only finding cancers that were problematic, explains Dr. Welch, the number of new prostate cancer cases would have stayed the same in the early 1990's after the test was introduced. But instead, the number of diagnosed cancer cases skyrocketed, and the rate is still higher than it used to be. "It looks more like a stock market graph than a graph of cancer biology," says

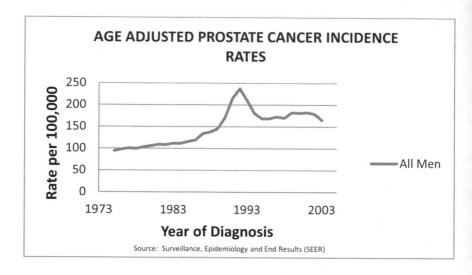

AGE ADJUSTED PROSTATE CANCER INCIDENCE RATES

Source: Surveillance, Epidemiology and End Results (SEER)

Welch. "These are the most erratic graphs in cancer anywhere."[11]

As a consequence of using the PSA test to detect prostate cancer, as many as 85% of men diagnosed with the disease don't have anything that will ever kill or even harm them at all.[12,13] What they have shouldn't even be called cancer and tragically, many end up receiving unnecessary cancer treatments which often result in severe, life-changing side effects or death.

A BIG PRICE TO PAY

During a prostate biopsy, a urologist will stick an 18-gauge needle through a man's rectal wall into his prostate gland 6 to 12 times, punching out core tissues for examination. It's well-established that biopsies suppress the immune system and promote cancer metastasis,[14-17] but there are a number of other reasons why a man might want to avoid a prostate biopsy.

A biopsy of the prostate can cause residual pain, blood in the urine, rectal bleeding,[18] erectile dysfunction,[19] and life-threatening infections.[20,21] This is probably because the biopsy needle first enters the rectum before piercing through the rectal wall into the prostate, which drags bacteria and fecal matter along with it. "The risk of hospitalization within 30 days of prostate biopsy was significantly higher than in a control population."[22] But the damage caused by punching holes in the prostate is minor compared to irradiating or surgically removing the prostate.

The two most common complications associated with having the prostate gland irradiated or removed are involuntary urination (urinary incontinence) and erectile dysfunction. *The New England Journal of Medicine* published a study in 2013 reporting that erectile dysfunction was "nearly universal" in patients 15 years after treatment for prostate cancer; "87.0% of those in the prostatectomy group and 93.9% of those in the radiotherapy group reporting an inability to achieve an erection sufficient for intercourse." Furthermore, all men experienced a decline in urinary continence that worsened as time went on. Some men had to wear diapers to prevent urinary leakage for the full 15-year follow-up period and probably for the rest of their lives.[23]

Despite the fact that the PSA test cannot detect prostate cancer and the extraordinary risk of a man having his sexuality and dignity stolen as a consequence of the test, almost 66% of men who undergo the PSA test are not even aware they've had it done;[24] their doctors simply do it as part of their routine physical, without their consent and without telling them the potential implications.[25]

MAMMOGRAPHY: BREAST CANCER SCREENING

First introduced in the 1970's,[26] mammography is an x-ray procedure that captures a photograph of the human breast used to detect breast cancer. While those who are invested in expensive mammography machinery or who rely on breast cancer screening to earn a living will assure you that mammography reduces breast cancer death rates, a number of large-scale studies have demonstrated that mammography provides no mortality benefit.[27-29]

A CLOSER LOOK...

The *Canadian National Breast Screening Study 1* involved 50,000 women aged 40 to 49 years and compared women who received 5 years of annual mammography screening and physical breast examinations with women who received only one physical breast examination. The study found that five annual mammograms and breast examinations in women aged 40 to 49 caused "no reduction in breast cancer mortality."[27]

The *Canadian National Breast Screening Study 2* involved 40,000 women aged 50 to 59 years and compared women who received five years of physical breast exams and mammography screening with women who received physical examinations only. The study concluded that in women aged 50 to 59, "the addition of annual mammography screening to physical examination has no impact on breast cancer mortality."[28]

The 25-year combined follow-up of the *Canadian National Breast Screening Study 1 and 2* was one of the largest and most meticulous studies ever conducted on mammography. Published in the *British Medical Journal* in 2014, results showed that "Annual mammography in women aged 40-59 does not reduce mortality from breast cancer beyond that of physical examination..."[29]

OVERDIAGNOSIS AND OVERTREATMENT

One of the major failures of mammography is how frequently it results in misdiagnosis of breast cancer. Over the course of 10 mammograms, women in the United States have between a 58-77% chance of being falsely diagnosed with breast cancer.[30] Another study found that for women with multiple breast cancer risk factors, like a strong family history, prolonged use of the contraceptive pill, etc. – the ones most strongly urged to have annual mammograms – the 10-year cumulative risk of being falsely diagnosed is "as high as 100 percent."[31] And of course, most will end up undergoing unnecessary treatments and suffering the horrendous side effects and mutilations associated with surgery and radiotherapy.

A 2012 study published in the *New England Journal of Medicine* concluded that one in three women (33%) diagnosed with breast cancer from a mammogram are misdiagnosed, and that a whopping 1.3 million women have been overdiagnosed by mammography in the past 30 years.[32]

A BIG PRICE TO PAY

Although the PSA test and mammography both fail to achieve their intended purpose of prolonging life, the PSA test involves only a blood sample while mammography exposes patients to damaging ionizing radiation and other harmful procedures.

First, the breast is tightly (and often painfully[33]) compressed between two imaging plates. If cancer is present in the breast during this compression it can result in metastasis.[34] Next, the x-ray image is taken and the patient receives a 10 mSv (millisievert) dose of ionizing radiation, approximately "1000 times greater than that from a chest x-ray," according to Dr. Samuel Epstein.[35]

THE DANGERS OF LOW-DOSE IONIZING RADIATION

The US government has long-held the position that low-doses of ionizing radiation are not hazardous to human health,[36] but since the early 1950's scientific research has indicated repeatedly that low-doses of radiation, like those administered to patients during x-ray imaging, do in fact cause increased rates of cancer.[37-53]

A Closer Look...

Researchers from the University of California investigated the relationship between x-ray exposure early in life and childhood leukemia in 2010. "Exposure to post-natal diagnostic X-rays is associated with increased risk of childhood ALL [acute childhood leukemia], the study concluded."[53]

A 1981 study published in *The Lancet* looked at cancer incidence in female factory workers who had been producing paint containing the radioactive element radium. The workers received radiation doses of 1-4mGy (milligray) per week and the study found, "Those in the group who were under 30 years of age when they started work show a significantly increased risk of dying from breast cancer."[46]

In 1989, scientists from Atlanta, Georgia investigated 1,030 women with scoliosis who had received multiple x-rays during childhood. Published in *The Journal of the National Cancer Institute*, at an average follow-up of 26 years, the study found an 83% greater incidence of cancer in the women compared to the general population. Importantly, their rate of cancer actually increased with time; women assessed more than 30 years later had a 140% greater incidence of cancer than the general population.[43]

LOW DOSES WORSE THAN HIGHER DOSES

Groundbreaking research, mostly on atomic bomb survivors and nuclear workers, is beginning to uncover a startling detail – not only are low doses of ionizing radiation enough to cause cancer, but low doses can actually be *more harmful* than larger ones.[54-57] E.B. Burlakova, director of the Radiobiology Committee of the Russian Academy of Sciences, has published a number of studies showing that the true dose-response of ionizing radiation is *biphasic*, meaning the damage increases from zero dose and then falls and then increases again.[58]

A CLOSER LOOK...

A 2008 study from Japan compared cancer prevalence in Hiroshima atomic bomb survivors with an unexposed population. The study found a significantly elevated risk of cancer in the exposed population, "Even at low and very low dose categories."[56]

Italian researchers exposed a group of mice to 1 Gy (gray) of ionizing radiation and another group of mice to 0.1 Gy of ionizing radiation and compared the effects. Results were published in the International Journal of Radiation Biology in 2008 and found, "In mice exposed to 1 Gy genetic damage was initially high and decreased during the experimental-time, while in the 0.1 Gy group damage, at first low, persisted and slightly increased."[54]

In 2016, researchers from Germany and Latvia questioned the validity of the current worldwide radiation risk model by investigating the genetic risks of exposure to low doses of radiation. The study found that, "Nearly all types of hereditary defects were found at doses as low as one to 10 mSv" and concluded that the current worldwide risk model for genetic effects of ionizing radiation is unsafe. Importantly, their work "supports a dose response relationship which is non-linear and is either biphasic or supralinear (hogs-back) and largely either saturates or falls above 10 mSv."[57]

How can a lower dose of ionizing radiation be *more* harmful than a larger dose? "Cancer arises when the DNA in cells is damaged, but the cells are not killed. Higher radiation doses are more likely to kill cells outright. So the lower doses are disproportionately carcinogenic," explains scientist Dr. Chris Busby.[59]

I asked Dr. Ray Peat the same question and he wrote, "The greatest effect per dose at low doses is sort of analogous to a car getting good gas mileage at low speeds with low wind resistance, compared to poor gas mileage at 80 to 100 mph, with considerable wind resistance. It isn't surprising if you think in terms of 'relatively mild electronic excitation,' producing chronic inflammatory signals, rather than all-or-nothing mutagenic events."

IS X-RAY IMAGING WORTH THE RISK?

A number of outspoken scientists have come to some startling conclusions regarding the use of medical imaging that the world needs to know about.

In 1971, Dr. Robert W. Gibson and his colleagues at the University of Buffalo conducted a study on the health effects of low-dose radiation from x-ray imaging. The researchers concluded that undergoing less than a dozen routine medical x-rays to the same part of the body increases the risk of leukemia by *at least* 60%.[60]

Dr. Irwin Bross headed the Tri-State Leukemia Study in the 1970's to determine what had been causing the alarming increases in leukemia at the time. The experiment included 16 million people from New York, Maryland, and Minnesota, and after exploring wide-ranging factors - including health history, occupational history, residential history, family background, cause of death for parents and grandparents, exposure to farm animals, pet ownership, whether or not the pets had ever been sick - Dr. Bross concluded that medical radiation in the form of diagnostic medical x-rays was *the main cause* of the rising rates of leukemia.[61]

Dr. John Gofman, medical physicist from the University of California, became a spokesman for the United States Atomic Energy Commission in the 1940's and spent almost 30 years travelling around glorifying the use of x-rays and other forms of radiation while denying that ionizing radiation had any harmful effects. Then, right in the middle of one of his speeches in the late 1960's, he realized that what he had been saying for three decades was insane:

"The big moment in my life happened while I was giving a health lecture to nuclear engineers. In the middle of my talk it hit me! What the hell am I saying? If you don't know whether low doses are safe or not, going ahead is exactly wrong. At that moment, I changed my position entirely."

Dr. Gofman suddenly went from being a government and nuclear industry 'talking head' to one of their biggest threats and soon found himself campaigning against the use of nuclear and medical x-ray technologies as well as writing a number of groundbreaking books.

The most significant conclusion made by Dr. Gofman after a lifetime of investigation into the biological effects of low-dose x-ray radiation was that accumulated radiation exposure from medical diagnostics is *the main cause* of over 50% of cancer deaths, 60% of heart disease deaths and over 80% of breast cancer deaths in the United States. While Dr. Gofman acknowledged other causes of cancer such as smoking, poor food quality and environmental toxins, he maintained that more than half the deaths from cancer and heart disease would not have occurred if it weren't for medical x-rays.[62]

Of course, none of the evidence above can be officially acknowledged or it would mean the death of the entire nuclear industry: power, weapons and medical imaging.

CANCER SCREENING: A PUBLIC HEALTH DISASTER

If mammography reveals an abnormality that the doctor suspects might be cancer, a biopsy will be performed. And if the biopsy reveals what the doctor interprets to be cancer, the woman suddenly becomes a breast cancer patient and will receive the whole works - surgery, chemotherapy and radiotherapy.

Despite evidence showing that surgical removal of one or both breasts (mastectomy) results in increased tumor recurrences and higher mortality,[63] or at best provides no additional benefit,[64] mastectomies have been on the rise in recent years.[65]

A CLOSER LOOK...

A 1995 study published in the *New England Journal of Medicine* followed up with breast cancer patients 10-years after receiving a mastectomy (surgical removal of one or both breasts) or a simple lumpectomy (surgical removal of only the tumor and some surrounding tissue) followed by whole-breast irradiation. Patients who received the mastectomy had more tumor recurrences and higher mortality 10-years following treatment than those who received the less invasive lumpectomy.[63]

This trend has a lot to do with the dramatic increase in biased media coverage of celebrity mastectomies since 2004, wrote scientists from the University of Michigan.

"The surgical treatment was significantly more likely to be mentioned [in the media] when a celebrity had bilateral mastectomies than unilateral mastectomy or breast conservation," their study concluded.[66]

One of the side effects a surgeon will probably fail to mention before performing a mastectomy is the subsequent almost-universal decline in self-esteem that women experience following the procedure.[67,68] "Patients who had had a mastectomy felt less attractive, less sexually desirable, and more ashamed of their breasts. They also experienced less enjoyment in their sexual relationships than they had before treatment."[69] To combat this hopelessness, many women return to their surgeons for breast implants, which unfortunately, only make a bad situation worse; as breast implants following mastectomy have been associated with a 3-fold increase in the risk of suicide.[70]

Now we return to our original question from the beginning of this chapter: does early detection and treatment of cancer save lives?

We've examined a number of studies showing that neither the PSA test nor mammography provide any mortality benefit whatsoever to the men and women who undergo them. Rather than saving lives, the widespread implementation of prostate and breast cancer screening has only enhanced the amount of men and women diagnosed and treated for cancer.

While this is obviously a lucrative and rewarding situation for the cancer industry, the mass overdiagnosis and overtreatment that sustains the booming cancer business comes at a considerable price; it means patients are frequently told they have cancer when they don't, and are frequently treated aggressively for diseases they don't have.

Maybe this is why Dr. Dean Burk once said of the American Cancer Society, "They lie like scoundrels," or why Dr. James Watson, the man who discovered DNA, declared before the California Assembly Committee of Health in 1976, "The American public is being sold a nasty bill of goods about cancer... Today, the press releases coming out of the National Cancer Institute have all the honesty of the Pentagon's."

TIMELESS QUOTES

"It is utter nonsense to claim that catching cancer symptoms early enough will increase the patient's chances of survival: not one scientist or study has proven that in any way."
- Dr. Hardin B. Jones

"There is simply no evidence that early detection of prostate cancer improves the health of patients."
- Dr. Steven H. Woolf, science advisor for US Preventive Services Task Force

"We're going to look back at this century and we're going to laugh eventually, but we'll cry first. This is one of the most barbaric periods. It's going to be called the Dark Ages of Medicine."
- Dr. Richard Shulze

CHAPTER 5

THE BATTLE FOR TRUTH

A MONUMENTAL RULING was made in US federal court in 2006 when a judge declared cigarette manufacturers *guilty* of conspiracy, fraud and racketeering. "They knew that cigarettes caused cancer, and they lied about it. They knew that nicotine was addictive, and they lied about that, too. They manipulated the levels of nicotine in cigarettes to sustain a smoker's addiction. And they denied that, knowing that that was incorrect. They lied about marketing to youth," said Dr. David Kessler, the government's lead witness in the case.[1]

By now, it shouldn't come as a surprise to most people that the tobacco industry engaged in conspiracy to sell their harmful products - but what might be surprising is that despite 100 million cigarette-induced deaths in the 20th century,[2] the judge imposed only minor penalties against the companies with "no hard hits on their wallets," reported the *Los Angeles Times*.[3]

THE PSYCHOLOGY OF THE RICH

For most of us, the idea of murdering over 100 million people for the sake of profit is incomprehensible. Scientists analyzing this bewildering psychology for a number of decades have come to the conclusion that higher social class "predicts increased unethical behavior."[4-6] A 2012 review on the subject noted that upper-class individuals were more likely to break the law, steal, lie, endorse unethical behavior and cheat to increase their chances of winning a prize.

With a $35 billion dollar annual 'prize' at stake for the tobacco industry,[7] perhaps now we can begin to understand the motivation behind their dreadful conduct, and also why the cancer industry - with its $125 billion dollar annual 'prize' - might be guilty of similar crimes.

THE CANCER INDUSTRY'S BAG OF TRICKS

There are a number of simple schemes used by the cancer industry to increase profits and a number that have taken greater effort to orchestrate. Starting simple, a 2015 study found that between the years 1995 to 2013, the average launch price of new cancer drugs increased by an average of $8,500 (10%) per year.[8] Some of the newest cancer drugs can cost patients over $150,000 USD for one year of treatment.[9]

- Have the production costs of these new drugs increased? No.

- Are they more effective? No.

- Pharmaceutical companies charge more for cancer drugs merely because they can.

Another trick used to boost chemotherapy drug earnings was exposed in a 2016 study titled *Overspending driven by oversized single dose vials of cancer drugs.*[10] Simply by selling one-size-fits-all vials of chemotherapy containing far more than what most patients need, an additional $3 billion is generated every year pushing product that ends up not being used.

SUPPRESSED CANCER CURES?

Most people I've talked to suspect the cancer industry has been involved in suppressing cancer cures from the public. From armed raids on the *Burzynski cancer clinic* in Texas to the political extinguishing of Renee Caisse's cancer clinic in Canada to the incredible story of Krebiozen – the active suppression of medicines that have threatened the profits of the cancer establishment have not been uncommon. One of the most fascinating accounts comes to us from Dr. Stan Monteith, who recently unlocked a story through the freedom of information act that had been hidden from the public for over 50 years.

In the 1950's, a man named Charles Tobey Jr. was diagnosed with cancer and told he had less than two years to live. But instead of submitting to the toxic orthodox cancer treatments that were recommended to him by his doctors, Tobey Jr. discovered an alternative approach that he opted for instead. The treatment was known as *The Lincoln Treatment*.

Developed by physician Dr. Robert Lincoln of Medford, Massachusetts, the Lincoln treatment consisted of taking viral and bacterial samples from patients, culturing them and then administering them back to patients through a nebulizer. Dr. Lincoln never charged more than $5 for the treatment and according to Tobey Jr. it was curative for many patients. "I saw hundreds of people who were getting well; I saw hundreds of husbands and wives who felt that they had new hope, and felt they were going to some one who was honestly trying to help them." Tobey Jr. underwent the Lincoln treatment, experienced a full recovery from cancer and credits the treatment for saving his life.[11]

After hearing that his son was cancer free and watching U.S. health authorities refuse to investigate the Lincoln treatment, his father – the prominent U.S. Senator Charles Toby - launched an official investigation into the cancer establishment. For the position, Toby appointed investigator Benedict Fitzgerald of the US Interstate Commerce Commission. His findings, titled *The Fitzgerald Report*, were presented to the U.S. senate in 1953, but the senate took no action and the inquest was never made

public.[12]   Here are some conclusions from his investigation, finally made public in 2007:

"My investigation to date should convince this committee
that a conspiracy does exist to stop the free flow and use
of drugs in interstate commerce which allegedly has solid
therapeutic value. Public and private funds have been
thrown around like confetti at a country fair to close up
and destroy clinics, hospitals, and scientific research
laboratories which do not conform to the viewpoint of
medical associations.

There is reason to believe that the AMA [American
Medical Association] has been hasty, capricious, arbitrary,
and outright dishonest...in an interstate conspiracy of
alarming proportions. Behind and over all this is the
weirdest conglomeration of corrupt motives, intrigue,
selfishness, jealousy, obstruction and conspiracy that I
have ever seen."
- Benedict F. Fitzgerald, Jr.

FRAUDULENT CANCER RESEARCH?

One of the schemes used by the tobacco industry to
mislead the American public about the safety of cigarettes
was they paid scientists to fabricate evidence declaring
cigarettes weren't harmful.[13] Is it possible that the cancer
industry too has been involved in fabricating scientific
evidence to misrepresent the safety and efficacy of its
cancer screening tools or treatments?

One study cited repeatedly by the industry in recent years as 'the perfect example' of the benefits of mammography was conducted in Denmark and published in 2005. Looking at the effects of mammography screening on women from Copenhagen for the first 10 years after it had been introduced in 1991, the study reported that mammography decreased mortality by 25%.[14]

However, in 2010, scientists from the Nordic Cochrane Centre in Denmark re-analyzed this group's findings and came to some startling conclusions. By expanding the scope of the study to include breast cancer mortality data from 10 years before screening was introduced and 10 years after screening was in practice in areas that weren't using screening, they discovered significant flaws in the original work. Published in the *British Medical Journal*, the study concluded that breast cancer actually slightly *increased* as a result of mammography screening.[15]

With an estimated 48 million mammograms performed in the United States every year,[17] at prices ranging from $43 to $1,989 for the test,[18] mammography represents between $2 billion and $91 billion dollars in annual revenue for the cancer industry, let alone the treatments that follow.

I contacted the Nordic Cochrane Centre and asked them if they knew of any industry funding behind this original work. They replied, "No industry funding of the

BMJ-study you refer to. The problem is intellectual bias, which is sometimes a problem of similar magnitude."

What the cancer industry did do in this case was exploit flawed research to sell a service that often causes unnecessary mutilation and increased death – which is no less immoral. There are a number of other studies that may have been funded by the industry to deliberately confuse the issue of mammography's safety and effectiveness. I'll present them and we can let the judge decide.

One of the most damning studies ever conducted on cancer screening and treatment was published in the journal *Medical Hypotheses* in 1996.[16] For the study, scientists re-examined 7 randomized mammography screening trials commonly cited as having produced evidence for reduced breast cancer mortality in order to resolve opposing claims about whether or not lives are saved through early detection. Their conclusions were as follows:

Early detection:
"No correlation was found between reduced breast cancer mortality and earlier surgical intervention. In fact, the trial with the most earlier surgical intervention had the smallest reduction in mortality; and that with the least earlier surgical intervention had the largest reduction in mortality. This demonstrates that the earlier-diagnosis hypothesis is invalid."

Cancer surgery:
"The conclusion from the previous analysis, that

surgery has not been shown to reduce mortality for any form of cancer, is therefore still valid."

Radiotherapy:

"Some correlation was established between reduced mortality and reduced use of radiotherapy…"

While inspecting the 7 mammography screening trials, researchers identified up to five factors that were variable in each trial, confounding the results. The reduction in deaths attributed to mammographic screening in the 7 trials resulted from the use of flawed statistical data that had reclassified a number of breast cancer deaths "as deaths from other causes following ischaemic heart damage caused by radiotherapy." In other words, people who were killed by radiotherapy treatment following early detection with mammography were labeled dead for reasons other than breast cancer, creating the false appearance of reduced breast cancer deaths and thus, the false appearance of a mortality benefit from both treatment and screening. Sound familiar?

You'll recall from the radiotherapy chapter, as first exposed by Dr. Ralph Moss, that official cancer mortality statistics have been altered to make it appear that cancer treatments are more effective than they actually are.[19-22]

By setting up a system where cancer mortality statistics are generated using death certificates, the stage was set so that even unbiased scientists would draw favorable conclusions for the ineffectual cancer screening programs and orthodox treatments; concealing the truth about their dangers and temporarily circumventing the cancer industry's inevitable collapse.

THE BATTLE FOR TRUTH

The unceasing battle being waged before us is one between individuals seeking empirical truth and those seeking monetary gain. The way people and organizations respond to criticisms of cancer screening tools and treatments reveals which side they are on.

When the U.S. Preventive Services Task Force publically recommended against PSA screening in 2011 "with moderate to high certainty" that its harms outweigh its benefits, the urology community - who rely on the steady influx of mostly-misdiagnosed prostate cancer patients provided by the PSA test to stay in business - fought back.

But instead of searching for flaws in the evidence used by the Task Force to make their recommendation, the urology community responded emotionally, calling their decision "cynical," "wreckless," and "unconscionable."[23] Skip Lockwood, CEO of the non-profit prostate cancer organization ZERO even went as far as saying their decision would amount to a death sentence for thousands of men each year. "The decision of no confidence on the PSA test by the U.S. government condemns tens of thousands of men to die this year and every year going forward..."[24]

Dr. Peter Gotzsche, leading Danish professor, statistician and head of the Nordic Cochrane Center, has been studying mammography for over two decades. Not only do mammograms do little to reduce death from breast cancer, but because women haven't been told the truth about the risks of mammography, he explains, some endure painful disfigurement and completely unnecessary treatment that may have shortened their lives.[25]

In 2000, Dr. Gotzsche and his colleague conducted a meta-analysis of eight randomized trials on mammography screening.[26] All six trials that had reported a mortality benefit from screening were found to have imbalances or inconsistencies in the way they were randomized, and of the two remaining trials that had been randomized adequately, neither reported a mortality benefit, prompting researchers to conclude, "Screening for breast cancer with mammography is unjustified." The study was published in *The Lancet* and its results generated a furious response.

In typical fashion of an industry fighting for its existence, the profiteers of mammography and breast cancer treatment didn't challenge the validity of Dr. Gotzsche's findings, but instead chose to attack him personally. "Often the attacks didn't even challenge my research - they were simply personal. I was said to be ignorant, careless and on a crusade against screening," said Gotzsche. Industry 'experts' urged women to ignore the report, government 'authorities' claimed there was no evidence behind it and Laszlo Tabar — author of one of the trials analyzed in the study — branded Gotzsche a 'woman hater.'[25]

The backlash against scientists reporting the ineffectiveness and dangers of cancer screening and treatments represents a desperate struggle by those who profit from cancer screening and treatment to prevent the public from realizing their greatest fear: *we are better off without them.*

MANY 'CANCERS' NOT EVEN HARMFUL

In a 2016 study published in the *Journal of the American Medical Association,* an international panel of doctors declared that a type of thyroid cancer, called Encapsulated Follicular Variant of Papillary Thyroid Carcinoma, is no longer cancer.[27] Although these tumors have been diagnosed as cancer and treated for decades, they have been found to never actually produce symptoms or any problems at all for patients when left untreated.

The push for reclassification began after Dr. Yuri E. Nikiforov from the University of Pittsburgh was asked his opinion about a small thyroid tumor in a 19-year-old woman. "I told the surgeon, who was a good friend, 'This is a very low grade tumor. You do not have to do anything else.'" But the surgeon replied that guidelines mandate she must remove the woman's entire thyroid gland and treat her with radioactive iodine. "I said, 'That's enough. Someone has to take responsibility and stop this madness.'"

As a result of Dr. Nikiforov's successful initiative, "...thousands of patients will be spared removal of their thyroid, treatment with radioactive iodine and regular checkups for the rest of their lives..." reported the *New York Times.*[28] But this particular type of thyroid tumor is not the only type of cancer that is harmless and in need of reclassification.

PROSTATE CANCER

The most astounding thing about the worldwide trillion-dollar[29] prostate cancer industry is that, even without treatment, almost no men diagnosed with prostate cancer will die from the disease.

In 1992, researchers followed up with untreated prostate cancer patients 10 years after they were diagnosed to determine their rate of survival. Results showed that only 8.5% of patients had died of prostate cancer. Some of the patients died of other causes but the overall survival rate of untreated prostate cancer patients at 10 years was almost 90%.[30] **But there's a catch:** some of the patients were given the hormone estrogen as treatment, which was probably rationalized by the mistaken belief that prostate cancer is caused by testosterone.[31,74-77] Since estrogen is officially classified a carcinogen, the 10-year survival rate of untreated prostate cancer patients - who are not given estrogen - is likely even greater. I searched for more studies on long-term survival rates of untreated prostate cancer patients and found the following.

In 2010, Swedish researchers published a study in the *Journal of the National Cancer Institute* that looked at how many men with untreated prostate cancer actually died from it. 10-years after being diagnosed with early-stage prostate cancer, results showed that only 2.4% of men died from the disease.[32]

"Of all the men diagnosed each year with prostate cancer, their lifetime risk of death from the disease is only 3 percent, which means, of course, that a man has 97% chance of surviving a diagnosis of prostate cancer..." explains Dr. Richard Ablin.

Because of the misuse of a simple test, millions of men have been shelling out $20,000-$50,000 or more[33] for treatments that have left them impotent and having to wear diapers - sometimes for the rest of their lives - all to treat a 'cancer' that was never even a threat.

BREAST CANCER

More than 60,000 women in the United States are diagnosed every year with a type of early-stage breast cancer called ductal carcinoma in situ (DCIS). [34] Between the years 1983 and 2003 there was a 500% increase in the number of women diagnosed with DCIS,[35] most of whom underwent damaging and unnecessary surgical procedures.[36] And in similar fashion to prostate cancer, virtually no women diagnosed with DCIS will die if their 'cancer' is left untreated.[27,39]

A study published in the *Journal of the American Medical Association* in 2015 investigated the 20-year mortality rates of more than 108,196 women diagnosed with ductal carcinoma in situ. Results showed that 20-years after diagnosis, treated or not, only 3.3% of the women died of breast cancer.[37]

The results of this study prompted Laura Esserman, M.D., and her colleague Christina Yau, Ph.D., from the

University of California to write an editorial, in which they stated, "Given the low breast cancer mortality risk, we should stop telling women that DCIS is an emergency and that they should schedule definitive surgery within 2 weeks of diagnosis."[38] While women diagnosed with DCIS are routinely frightened into quickly undergoing treatment, this study suggests the best treatment for these patients is no treatment.

NUMEROUS OTHER CANCERS

One of Dr. Peter Gotzsche's critical messages is that many of the occult tumors detected during breast[39] and prostate cancer screening[40] may never become advanced enough to harm patients. As a result, thousands of people who would have remained perfectly healthy – because their cancers would have never caused a problem – become cancer patients.

"It is a biological fact of life that we cannot avoid getting cancer as we get older," says Dr. Gotzsche. "It's so common nearly all middle-aged people will have some sign of it and most of them will die without having had any symptoms as a result."[25]

For years, many cancer experts have been calling for the reclassification of small cancers of the breast and prostate, lung, brain, thyroid, skin and kidney.[27] A growing body of experiments conducted by forward-thinking scientists are showing that when we avoid harming the body with destructive treatments, many cancers may ultimately undergo spontaneous regression.

SPONTANEOUS REGRESSION OF CANCER

Spontaneous regression, or the complete disappearance of cancer in the absence of treatment, was first documented in the medical literature in 1742.[41] Since then, spontaneous regression has been documented in virtually every type of cancer; including breast,[42] prostate,[43] sarcoma,[44] seminoma,[45] melanoma,[46] basal cell carcinoma,[46] leukemia,[47] stomach,[48] kidney,[47] colon,[49] cervical,[50] liver,[51] lung[51] and brain.[52]

In the early to mid-1900's, the frequency of spontaneous regression of cancer was believed to be 1 in 80,000-100,000 patients,[61] but modern research is showing that spontaneous regression is vastly more common. "One of the reasons that spontaneous regression of tumors seems so rare is undoubtedly that most tumors are quickly cut out by surgeons," wrote Dr. Ray Peat.

When patients aren't scared-to-death and rushed into treatment by their doctors, rates of spontaneous regression can be seen as high as 7% in renal carcinoma patients,[62] up to 15% in melanoma patients[63] and up to 20% in patients with low-grade lymphoma.[64] Some studies have recorded even higher rates of spontaneous regression.[65-68]

A CLOSER LOOK...

A 1984 study from the New England Journal of Medicine examined survival rates of 83 untreated cancer patients with advanced non-Hodgkin's lymphoma. Results showed that 83% of patients were alive at 5-years and 73% were still alive at 10-years and remarkably, "Spontaneous regressions occurred in 19 untreated patients (23 percent)."[65]

A 2008 American study examined the prevalence of invasive breast cancer in 100,000 women who received either mammography screening or no screening. The first group was screened every two years (receiving six more mammograms per woman on average) and the control group underwent a single screening at the end of their six-year observation period to assess for cancer. At the end of the six-years, the study found that 22% more women in the screening group had invasive breast cancer than the control group - suggesting that 22% of cancers detected by repeated mammographic screening had spontaneously regressed in the absence of screening. In other words, by simply avoiding the repeated doses of ionizing radiation administered during mammography, the body is given a chance to heal on its own; and often it does.[66]

In 1997, scientists from the Royal Prince Alfred Hospital in Australia looked at the prevalence of spontaneous regression in skin tumors. Published in *The Australasian Journal of Dermatology*, the study found that 25% of melanomas and 50% of basal cell carcinomas spontaneously regressed on their own. Additionally, in two other types of skin tumors called keratoacanthoma and epithelioma, "nearly all the tumours regress completely."[67]

A number of studies have suggested that spontaneous regression is mediated by the body's immune system;[53-60]

"Analysis of the regressing tumors revealed heavy infiltration by T lymphocytes as compared to non-regressing tumors," concluded scientists from Kuwait University in 2005.[60]

Given that only about 2 percent of patients survive 5-years following chemotherapy, simply by rejecting harmful orthodox cancer treatments, survival rates can be increased by 5-times, 10-times, even 25-times. Now, imagine the prospect of survival if the rejection of orthodox cancer treatments is accompanied by the use of medicines that are both safe and effective.

THE CANCER INDUSTRY'S BIGGEST SECRET

There's a reason why women and men are never fully-informed about the dangers and potential implications of mammography screening, PSA screening, surgery, chemotherapy or radiotherapy - because if they were, nobody would ever agree to undergo them.

Doctors see first hand that surgery, chemotherapy and radiotherapy commonly increase the rate of cancer metastasis 100-fold,[78] and that's why almost 90% of doctors have said they would refuse these treatments for themselves if they were terminally ill and dying.[79]

In the previous chapter, three large mammography screening trials, all of which reported no mortality benefits from mammography screening were presented. A closer look at the data from two of those studies reveals that mortality was actually *increased* in women who underwent mammography screening.[69,70]

A CLOSER LOOK...

At the 7-year follow-up for the *Canadian National Breast Screening Study 1,* researchers discovered a 36% *increased* mortality among women in the mammography screening group; "38 women in the mammography group and 28 women in the usual care group had died of breast cancer."[69]

At the 25-year follow-up of the *Canadian National Breast Screening Study* 1 and 2, researchers found that 180 women died of breast cancer in the mammography screening group and only 171 women in the control group.[70]

Another large-scale mammography study was The Malmö Mammographic Screening Trial of 1988. The Malmö study included over 40,000 women to determine whether repeated mammographic screening reduces mortality from breast cancer. At an average follow-up of 9 years, results showed that in women under the age of 55 who underwent mammography screening, breast cancer deaths *increased* by 29%.[71]

THE UNTREATED LIVE LONGER

In 1979, American Biologist Dr. Maurice Fox published an article in the *Journal of the American Medical Association* comparing survival rates of breast cancer patients treated using orthodox methods with those who were left untreated. After reviewing data from studies conducted at the Harvard School of Public Health, Dr. Fox concluded, "Those who refused medical procedures had a lower mortality rate than those who submitted."[72]

Dr. Hardin B. Jones, professor of medical physics at the University of California, Berkeley and leading US cancer statistician for over 30 years, sent shockwaves through a 1969 seminar for the American Cancer Society when he announced the results of his 25-year study[73] comparing survival rates of treated cancer patients with untreated cancer patients:

"My studies have proved conclusively that untreated cancer victims live up to four times longer than treated individuals. If one has cancer and opts to do nothing at all, he will live longer and feel better than if he undergoes radiation, chemotherapy or surgery, other than when used in immediate life-threatening situations."

In 1975, twice as many women were diagnosed with breast cancer than in 1935 and twice as many women died,[72] evidencing what appears to be the most vile, appalling and despicable truth those in the cancer industry have worked so diligently to conceal:

Cancer deaths have increased in parallel to the number of people treated.

TIMELESS QUOTES

"We have a multi-billion dollar industry that is killing people, right and left, just for financial gain."
- Dr. Glen Warner

"If I contracted cancer, I would never go to a standard cancer treatment centre. Cancer victims who live far from such centers have a chance."
- Professor Charles Mathe

"You see, it is not the cancer that kills the victim. It's the breakdown of the defense mechanism that eventually brings death. With every cancer patient who keeps in excellent physical shape and boosts his health to build up his natural resistance, there's a high chance that the body will find its own defense against cancer. He may have many good years left in good health. He shouldn't squander them by being made into a hopeless invalid through radical intervention which has zero chance of extending his life."
- Dr. Hardin B. Jones, Ph.D.,quoted at Midnight, September 1, 1975.

"It is better not to apply any treatment in cases of occult cancer; for if treated, the patients die quickly; but if not treated, they hold out for a long time."
- Hippocrates (460-370 BC)

"It is from nature that the disease comes, and from nature comes the cure, not from physicians."
- Paracelsus (1493-1541)

CONCLUSION

WHEN A HUMAN BEING is sick with cancer, they deserve the absolute safest and most effective medicines known to man. Period.

Yet in this world, cancer patients are routinely rushed into oncology centers where doctors sentence them to death using treatments that make industrial animal slaughterhouses look humane.

When somebody survives the total onslaught of surgery, chemotherapy and radiotherapy, they have not survived because these war weapons have somehow healed them; they have survived *despite* these so-called treatments because they are extraordinarily strong and have an unrelenting will to survive.

In writing this book I have come to the realization that what I had long suspected about my mother's death was in fact true: My mother didn't die of cancer. She was murdered-for-profit by an industry that cares more about making money than saving lives.

What else are we to expect from an enterprise claiming that butchering sick people with knives, poisoning them with mustard gas and burning them with ionizing radiation will improve their health?

The monstrous $126 billion dollar cancer industry, hell-bent on preserving its profits at any cost, continues its murderous rampage to this day. The mind of the beast wells up with excitement at the thought of 50% of all human beings alive being one day diagnosed with cancer. Only an informed population of people, willing to stand up for themselves and make their own health decisions, can put an end to the cancer industry's reign of terror.

With this raging bull charging directly at humanity the question remains: Are we going to continue letting the cancer industry annihilate us and everyone we love until there's no one left - or stand up for ourselves and watch this beast plummet into the eternal, fiery depths of hell?

THE CANCER INDUSTRY CRUMBLES

If our goal as a society is to reduce the suffering in this world and create better future for all human beings, then it's clear the present screening tests and treatments offered by the cancer industry must be banished from the Earth.

If you've decided there's no way in hell you'll ever submit to the cancer industry's diagnostic tests or its so-called treatments, then make that decision clear to yourself and to the people around you. Be vocal about it and speak the truth.

Never be afraid to assert yourself and say *'no'* to your doctor or anybody trying to sell you a product or service. Remember, it's your body and your choice.

This is literally all it will take in order for us to forever eliminate the insane practice of using weapons of war on the sickest among us. As with all products and services that go unpurchased, they will quickly cease being produced.

HEALING THE WORLD AND ENDING CANCER

Our chances of surviving a cancer diagnosis is increased 400% simply by saying *'no'* to useless cancer screening tests and mainstream cancer treatments like surgery, chemotherapy and radiotherapy. Now imagine our prognosis if we couple the elimination of these damaging treatments with protocols that address the root cause of the disease without side effects.

This is the next step in our investigation into cancer. Equally critical as understanding that the cancer industry is doing more harm than good is knowing what to replace that void with.

The goal of the next book in this *Curing Cancer Series* will be to finally solve some of the greatest mysteries of cancer, some of which have escaped scientists for centuries, including:

- What is cancer?

- What causes cancer?

- What is a tumor?

- What are the safest and most effective ways to remedy the root cause of cancer?

Thank you for reading this book. I hope you've learned many valuable things that will empower you to make your own decisions in health and in life. Be sure to share this book with someone you love.

REFERENCES

INTRODUCTION

1. The American Cancer Society. (2017). All Cancer Facts & Figures. Available: https://www.cancer.org/research/cancer-facts-statistics/all-cancer-facts-figures.html. [January 31, 2017].

2. Lizzie Parry. (2014). 'The war on cancer may NEVER be won': Cure 'could be impossible' because the disease is so highly evolved. Mail Online. Available: http://www.dailymail.co.uk/health/article-2731765/The-war-cancer-NEVER-won-Cure-impossible-disease-highly-evolved.html. [January 31, 2017].

3. Kelsey Campbell-Dollaghan. (2013). Infographic: How People Died In The 20th Century. Available: https://www.fastcodesign.com/1672161/infographic-how-people-died-in-the-20th-century. [January 31, 2017].

4. Mariotto AB, Yabroff KR, Shao Y, Feuer EJ, Brown ML. Projections of the cost of cancer care in the United States: 2010-2020. J Natl Cancer Inst. 2011;103(2):117-28.

5. GLOBAL NUCLEAR COVER UP: Ernest Sternglass. Berkeley, 2006. r3VOLt23. YouTube. Available: https://www.youtube.com/watch?v=CLw2ISdx9eo. [January 31, 2017].

6. The American Cancer Society medical and editorial content team. (2016). Lifetime Risk of Developing or Dying from Cancer. Available: http://www.cancer.org/cancer/cancerbasics/lifetime-probability-of-developing-or-dying-from-cancer. [January 31, 2017].

7. World Health Organization. Global cancer rates could increase by 50% to 15 million by 2020. Available: http://www.who.int/mediacentre/news/releases/200 3/pr27/en.[January 31, 2017].

SURGERY

1. Leape LL. Unnecessary surgery. Health Serv Res. 1989;24(3):351-407.

2. Rondberg, T.A. 1998. *Under the Influence of Modern Medicine.* Chiropractic Journal, 156 pps.

3.   Mendelsohn, R.S. 1979. *Confessions of a Medical Heretic.* McGraw-Hill Education, New York City, NY, 197 pps.

4.   Leape LL. Unnecessary surgery. Annu Rev Public Health. 1992;13:363-83.

5.   Eisler, P. and Hansen, B. (2013). *Doctors Perform Thousands of Unnecessary Surgeries.* USA Today. [Online.] Available: http://www.usatoday.com/story/news/nation/2013/06/18/unnecessary-surgery-usa-today-investigation/2435009 [December 1, 2016].

6.   Tayade MC, Dalvi SD. Fundamental Ethical Issues in Unnecessary Surgical Procedures. J Clin Diagn Res. 2016;10(4):JE01-4.

7.   Chisholm, D. (2016). *Many operations are no better than placebo, says top surgeon.* The Listener. [Online]. Available: http://www.noted.co.nz/health/health/many-operations-are-no-better-than-placebo-says-top-surgeon [December 1, 2016].

8.   Detre K, Murphy ML, Hultgren H. Effect of coronary bypass surgery on longevity in high and low risk patients. Report from the V.A. Cooperative Coronary Surgery Study. Lancet. 1977;2(8051):1243-5.

9.   Myocardial infarction and mortality in the coronary artery surgery study (CASS) randomized trial. N Engl J Med. 1984;310(12):750-8.

10.   Hueb W, Lopes NH, Gersh BJ, et al. Five-year follow-up of the Medicine, Angioplasty, or Surgery Study (MASS II): a randomized controlled clinical trial of 3

therapeutic strategies for multivessel coronary artery disease. Circulation. 2007;115(9):1082-9.

11. Texas Heart Institute (2016). *Limited-Access Heart Surgery.* [Online]. Available: [December 1, 2016].

12. Giacomino BD, Cram P, Vaughan-sarrazin M, Zhou Y, Girotra S. Association of Hospital Prices for Coronary Artery Bypass Grafting With Hospital Quality and Reimbursement. Am J Cardiol. 2016;117(7):1101-6.

13. Heaton JP, Evans H, Adams MA, Smith K, Morales A. Coronary artery bypass graft surgery and its impact on erectile function: a preliminary retrospective study. Int J Impot Res. 1996;8(1):35-9.

14. Dhein S, Grassl M, Gerdom M, et al. Organ-protective effects on the liver and kidney by minocycline in small piglets undergoing cardiopulonary bypass. Naunyn Schmiedebergs Arch Pharmacol. 2015;388(6):663-76.

15. Walter H. Walshe, The Anatomy, Physiology, Pathology and Treatment of Cancer, (Boston: Ticknor & Co., 1844).

16. Wilt TJ, Brawer MK, Jones KM, et al. Radical prostatectomy versus observation for localized prostate cancer. N Engl J Med. 2012;367(3):203-13.

17. Jacobson JA, Danforth DN, Cowan KH, et al. Ten-year results of a comparison of conservation with mastectomy in the treatment of stage I and II breast cancer. N Engl J Med. 1995;332(14):907-11.

18. Vila J, Gandini S, Gentilini O. Overall survival according to type of surgery in young (≤40 years) early breast cancer patients: A systematic meta-analysis

comparing breast-conserving surgery versus mastectomy. Breast. 2015;24(3):175-81.

19. Pin YK, Khoo K, Tham M, et al. Lymphadenectomy promotes tumor growth and cancer cell dissemination in the spontaneous RET mouse model of human uveal melanoma. Oncotarget. 2015;6(42):44806-18.

20. Langley RR, Fidler IJ. Tumor cell-organ microenvironment interactions in the pathogenesis of cancer metastasis. Endocr Rev. 2007;28(3):297-321.

21. Langley RR, Fidler IJ. The seed and soil hypothesis revisited--the role of tumor-stroma interactions in metastasis to different organs. Int J Cancer. 2011;128(11):2527-35.

22. Chen LL, Blumm N, Christakis NA, Barabási AL, Deisboeck TS. Cancer metastasis networks and the prediction of progression patterns. Br J Cancer. 2009;101(5):749-58.

23. Marie P, Clunet J. Fréquences des métastases viscérales chez les souris cancéreuses après ablation chirurgicale de leur tumeur. *Bull Assoc Franç pour l'étude du cancer* 1910;3:19-23.

24. Tyzzer EE. Factors in the production and growth of tumor metastases. J Med Res 1913;23:309-332.

25. Cole WH. Spontaneous regression of cancer: the metabolic triumph of the host?. Ann N Y Acad Sci. 1974;230:111-41.

26. Krokowski, E.H.: Is the Current Treatment of Cancer Self-Limiting in the Extent of its Success? J Int Acad Preventive Medicine, 6 (1) 23 – 39, 1979.

27. Retsky M, Demicheli R, Hrushesky W, Baum M, Gukas I. Surgery triggers outgrowth of latent distant disease in breast cancer: an inconvenient truth?. Cancers (Basel). 2010;2(2):305-37.

28. Lange PH, Hekmat K, Bosl G, Kennedy BJ, Fraley EE. Acclerated growth of testicular cancer after cytoreductive surgery. Cancer. 1980;45(6):1498-506.

29. Demicheli R, Retsky MW, Hrushesky WJ, Baum M. Tumor dormancy and surgery-driven interruption of dormancy in breast cancer: learning from failures. Nat Clin Pract Oncol. 2007;4(12):699-710.

30. Retsky MW, Demicheli R, Hrushesky WJ, Baum M, Gukas ID. Dormancy and surgery-driven escape from dormancy help explain some clinical features of breast cancer. APMIS. 2008;116(7-8):730-41.

31. Goldstein MR, Mascitelli L. Surgery and cancer promotion: are we trading beauty for cancer?. QJM. 2011;104(9):811-5.

32. Hanin L, Bunimovich-mendrazitsky S. Reconstruction of the natural history of metastatic cancer and assessment of the effects of surgery: Gompertzian growth of the primary tumor. Math Biosci. 2014;247:47-58.

33. Hanin L, Pavlova L. A quantitative insight into metastatic relapse of breast cancer. J Theor Biol. 2016;394:172-81.

34. Sano F, Ueda K, Murakami J, Hayashi M, Nishimoto A, Hamano K. Enhanced tumor growth in the remaining lung after major lung resection. J Surg Res. 2016;202(1):1-7.

35. Desborough JP. The stress response to trauma and surgery. Br J Anaesth. 2000;85(1):109-17.

36. Hooli 1 RS, Gavimath CC, Ravishankera BE. Study to assess stress among cardiac surgical patients. International Journal of Pharmaceutical Applications. 2012; Vol 3, Issue 1, 2012, pp 282-288.

37. Gibbs J, Cull W, Henderson W, Daley J, Hur K, Khuri SF. Preoperative Serum Albumin Level as a Predictor of Operative Mortality and MorbidityResults From the National VA Surgical Risk Study. *Arch Surg.* 1999;134(1):36-42.

38. Kim WK, Ke K, Sul OJ, et al. Curcumin protects against ovariectomy-induced bone loss and decreases osteoclastogenesis. J Cell Biochem. 2011;112(11):3159-66.

39. Yu EW, Bouxsein ML, Roy AE, et al. Bone loss after bariatric surgery: discordant results between DXA and QCT bone density. J Bone Miner Res. 2014;29(3):542-50.

40. Kronzer VL, Avidan MS. Preventing postoperative delirium: all that glisters is not gold. Lancet. 2016;388(10054):1854-1856.

41. Benson RA, Ozdemir BA, Matthews D, Loftus IM. A systematic review of postoperative cognitive decline following open and endovascular aortic aneurysm surgery. Ann R Coll Surg Engl. 2016;:1-4.

42. Fidalgo AR, Cibelli M, White JP, Nagy I, Maze M, Ma D. Systemic inflammation enhances surgery-induced cognitive dysfunction in mice. Neurosci Lett. 2011;498(1):63-6.

43. Kumar N, Singh JG. A study of surgical stress in female patients. Available: https://www.researchgate.net/publication/279471510 _A_study_of_Surgical_Stress_in_Female_patients [December 1, 2016].

44. Staff NP, Engelstad J, Klein CJ, et al. Post-surgical inflammatory neuropathy. Brain. 2010;133(10):2866-80.

45. Egido JA, Castillo O, Roig B, et al. Is psycho-physical stress a risk factor for stroke? A case-control study. J Neurol Neurosurg Psychiatr. 2012;83(11):1104-10.

46. Schachter SC. Iatrogenic seizures. Neurol Clin. 1998;16(1):157-70.

47. Perdrizet GA, Lena CJ, Shapiro DS, Rewinski MJ. Preoperative stress conditioning prevents paralysis after experimental aortic surgery: increased heat shock protein content is associated with ischemic tolerance of the spinal cord. J Thorac Cardiovasc Surg. 2002;124(1):162-70.

48. Fukuda M, Hirota M, Sato S. Bone lesions and dental caries after gastrectomy--evaluation of milk intolerance and operative procedure. Jpn J Surg. 1986;16(1):36-41.

49. Carr EC, Nicky thomas V, Wilson-barnet J. Patient experiences of anxiety, depression and acute pain after surgery: a longitudinal perspective. Int J Nurs Stud. 2005;42(5):521-30.

50. Thorell A, Nygren J, Ljungqvist O. Insulin resistance: a marker of surgical stress. Curr Opin Clin Nutr Metab Care. 1999;2(1):69-78.

51. Ramachandran A, Balasubramanian KA. Protease activation during surgical stress in the rat small intestine. J Surg Res. 2000;92(2):283-90.

52. Briusov PG, Osipov IS. [Stress ulcers of the gastrointestinal tract in surgical patients]. Voen Med Zh. 1998;319(1):30-8.

53. Martin LF, Booth FV, Reines HD, et al. Stress ulcers and organ failure in intubated patients in surgical intensive care units. Ann Surg. 1992;215(4):332-7.

54. Watters JM, Clancey SM, Moulton SB, Briere KM, Zhu JM. Impaired recovery of strength in older patients after major abdominal surgery. Ann Surg. 1993;218(3):380-90.

55. Pierce V, Kendrick P. Ischemic optic neuropathy after spine surgery. AANA J. 2010;78(2):141-5.

56. Wiener DJ, Rüfenacht S, Koch HJ, Mauldin EA, Mayer U, Welle MM. Estradiol-induced alopecia in five dogs after contact with a transdermal gel used for the treatment of postmenopausal symptoms in women. Vet Dermatol. 2015;26(5):393-6, e90-1.

57. West JM. Wound healing in the surgical patient: influence of the perioperative stress response on perfusion. AACN Clin Issues Crit Care Nurs. 1990;1(3):595-601.

58. Reversible sensorineural hearing loss after non-otological surgery under general anaesthetic. Postgraduate Medical Journal. 2000;76(895):304.

59. Badner NH, Knill RL, Brown JE, Novick TV, Gelb AW. Myocardial infarction after noncardiac surgery. Anesthesiology. 1998;88(3):572-8.

60. Nito I, Waspadji S, Harun S, Markum HM. Correlation between cortisol levels and myocardial infarction mortality among intensive coronary care unit patients during first seven days in hospital. Acta Med Indones. 2004;36(1):8-14.

61. Gallerani M, Maida G, Boari B, Galeotti R, Rocca T, Gasbarro V. High output heart failure due to an iatrogenic arterio-venous fistula after lumbar disc surgery. Acta Neurochir (Wien). 2007;149(12):1243-7.

62. Güder G, Bauersachs J, Frantz S, et al. Complementary and incremental mortality risk prediction by cortisol and aldosterone in chronic heart failure. Circulation. 2007;115(13):1754-61.

63. Xie ZB, Zhu SL, Peng YC, et al. Postoperative hepatitis B virus reactivation and surgery-induced immunosuppression in patients with hepatitis B-related hepatocellular carcinoma. J Surg Oncol. 2015;112(6):634-42.

64. Xu P, Zhang P, Sun Z, Wang Y, Chen J, Miao C. Surgical trauma induces postoperative T-cell dysfunction in lung cancer patients through the programmed death-1 pathway. Cancer Immunol Immunother. 2015;64(11):1383-92.

65. Goldfarb Y, Sorski L, Benish M, Levi B, Melamed R, Ben-eliyahu S. Improving postoperative immune status and resistance to cancer metastasis: a combined perioperative approach of immunostimulation and prevention of excessive surgical stress responses. Ann Surg. 2011;253(4):798-810.

66. Nakatani T, Kobayashi K. [Surgical stress and organ dysfunction: liver]. Nihon Geka Gakkai Zasshi. 1996;97(9):752-8.

67. Massard G, Wihlm JM. Postoperative atelectasis. Chest Surg Clin N Am. 1998;8(3):503-28, viii.

68. Mogos V, Mogos S. Iatrogenic erectile dysfunction after pelvic surgery: prostatectomy, colonic and rectal surgery. Available: https://www.researchgate.net/publication/267398060 _IATROGENIC_ERECTILE_DYSFUNCTION_A FTER_PELVIC_SURGERY_PROSTATECTOMY_ COLONIC_AND_RECTAL_SURGERY. [December 1, 2016].

69. Canbaz S, Ege T, Sunar H, Cikirikcioglu M, Acipayam M, Duran E. The effects of cardiopulmonary bypass on androgen hormones in coronary artery bypass surgery. J Int Med Res. 2002;30(1):9-14.

70. Yasuma F, Okada T. [Sleep disturbances complicated by surgical stress; a questionnaire survey of 50 patients]. Masui. 1989;38(1):66-70.

71. Gejrot T, Notter G. Effects of surgical stress on thyroid function in man. Acta Otolaryngol. 1962;55:1-10.

72. Li RL, Zhang ZZ, Peng M, et al. Postoperative impairment of cognitive function in old mice: a possible role for neuroinflammation mediated by HMGB1, S100B, and RAGE. J Surg Res. 2013;185(2):815-24.

73. Terrando N, Yang T, Wang X, et al. Systemic HMGB1 Neutralization Prevents Postoperative Neurocognitive

Dysfunction in Aged Rats. Front Immunol. 2016;7:441.

74. Helmy SA, Wahby MA, El-nawaway M. The effect of anaesthesia and surgery on plasma cytokine production. Anaesthesia. 1999;54(8):733-8.

75. Hildebrand F, Pape HC, Krettek C. [The importance of cytokines in the posttraumatic inflammatory reaction]. Unfallchirurg. 2005;108(10):793-4, 796-803.

76. Thaeter M, Knobe M, Vande kerckhove M, et al. Perioperative inflammatory response in major fracture: do geriatric patients behave differently?. Eur J Trauma Emerg Surg. 2016;42(5):547-551.

77. Cibelli M, Fidalgo AR, Terrando N, et al. Role of interleukin-1beta in postoperative cognitive dysfunction. Ann Neurol. 2010;68(3):360-8.

78. Sun L, Jia P, Zhang J, et al. Production of inflammatory cytokines, cortisol, and Aβ1-40 in elderly oral cancer patients with postoperative delirium. Neuropsychiatr Dis Treat. 2016;12:2789-2795.

79. Maniwa Y, Okada M, Ishii N, Kiyooka K. Vascular endothelial growth factor increased by pulmonary surgery accelerates the growth of micrometastases in metastatic lung cancer. Chest. 1998;114(6):1668-75.

80. Tagliabue E, Agresti R, Carcangiu ML, et al. Role of HER2 in wound-induced breast carcinoma proliferation. Lancet. 2003;362(9383):527-33.

81. Nguyen DP, Li J, Tewari AK. Inflammation and prostate cancer: the role of interleukin 6 (IL-6). BJU Int. 2014;113(6):986-92.

82. Kooguchi K, Kobayashi A, Kitamura Y, et al. Elevated expression of inducible nitric oxide synthase and inflammatory cytokines in the alveolar macrophages after esophagectomy. Crit Care Med. 2002;30(1):71-6.

83. Morbidelli L, Donnini S, Ziche M. Role of nitric oxide in the modulation of angiogenesis. Curr Pharm Des. 2003;9(7):521-30.

84. Morbidelli L, Donnini S, Ziche M. Role of nitric oxide in tumor angiogenesis. Cancer Treat Res. 2004;117:155-67.

85. Ziche M, Morbidelli L. Nitric oxide and angiogenesis. J Neurooncol. 2000;50(1-2):139-48.

86. Morbidelli L, Donnini S, Ziche M. Role of nitric oxide in tumor angiogenesis. Cancer Treat Res. 2004;117:155-67.

87. Gallo O, Masini E, Morbidelli L, et al. Role of nitric oxide in angiogenesis and tumor progression in head and neck cancer. J Natl Cancer Inst. 1998;90(8):587-96.

88. Vidal MJ, Zocchi MR, Poggi A, Pellegatta F, Chierchia SL. Involvement of nitric oxide in tumor cell adhesion to cytokine-activated endothelial cells. J Cardiovasc Pharmacol. 1992;20 Suppl 12:S155-9.

89. Klaunig JE, Kamendulis LM, Hocevar BA. Oxidative stress and oxidative damage in carcinogenesis. Toxicol Pathol. 2010;38(1):96-109.

90. Shavit Y, Weidenfeld J, Dekeyser FG, et al. Effects of surgical stress on brain prostaglandin E2 production and on the pituitary-adrenal axis: attenuation by

preemptive analgesia and by central amygdala lesion. Brain Res. 2005;1047(1):10-7.

91. Wolfle D. Enhancement of carcinogen-induced malignant cell transformation by prostaglandin F2a. 2003; Volume 188, Issues 2-3, pages 139-147.

92. Fabre B, Grosman H, Gonzalez D, et al. Prostate Cancer, High Cortisol Levels and Complex Hormonal Interaction. Asian Pac J Cancer Prev. 2016;17(7):3167-71.

93. Kim HM, Ha KS, Hwang IC, Ahn HY, Youn CH. Random Serum Cortisol as a Predictor for Survival of Terminally Ill Patients With Cancer: A Preliminary Study. Am J Hosp Palliat Care. 2016;33(3):281-5.

94. Cohen L, Cole SW, Sood AK, et al. Depressive symptoms and cortisol rhythmicity predict survival in patients with renal cell carcinoma: role of inflammatory signaling. PLoS ONE. 2012;7(8):e42324.

95. Schmidt M, Löffler G. Induction of aromatase in stromal vascular cells from human breast adipose tissue depends on cortisol and growth factors. FEBS Lett. 1994;341(2-3):177-81.

96. Wang WS, Liu C, Li WJ, Zhu P, Li JN, Sun K. Involvement of CRH and hCG in the induction of aromatase by cortisol in human placental syncytiotrophoblasts. Placenta. 2014;35(1):30-6.

97. Wang W, Li J, Ge Y, et al. Cortisol induces aromatase expression in human placental syncytiotrophoblasts through the cAMP/Sp1 pathway. Endocrinology. 2012;153(4):2012-22.

98. Women's Health Initiative. Available: https://www.nhlbi.nih.gov/whi/estro_alone.htm. [December 1, 2016].

99. Goldstein MR, Mascitelli L. Surgery and cancer promotion: are we trading beauty for cancer?. QJM. 2011;104(9):811-5.

100. Waters JH, Miller LR, Clack S, Kim JV. Cause of metabolic acidosis in prolonged surgery. Crit Care Med. 1999;27(10):2142-6.

101. Macniven E, Decatanzaro D, Younglai EV. Chronic stress increases estrogen and other steroids in inseminated rats. Physiol Behav. 1992;52(1):159-62.

102. Shavit Y, Weidenfeld J, Dekeyser FG, et al. Effects of surgical stress on brain prostaglandin E2 production and on the pituitary-adrenal axis: attenuation by preemptive analgesia and by central amygdala lesion. Brain Res. 2005;1047(1):10-7.

103. Singh, M. Stress response and anesthesia: Altering the peri and post-operative management. Indian J. Anaesth. 2003; 47 (6): 427-434.

104. Soll C, Jang JH, Riener MO, et al. Serotonin promotes tumor growth in human hepatocellular cancer. Hepatology. 2010;51(4):1244-54.

105. Gurbuz N, Ashour AA, Alpay SN, Ozpolat B. Down-regulation of 5-HT1B and 5-HT1D receptors inhibits proliferation, clonogenicity and invasion of human pancreatic cancer cells. PLoS ONE. 2014;9(8):e105245.

106. Pai VP, Marshall AM, Hernandez LL, Buckley AR, Horseman ND. Altered serotonin physiology in

human breast cancers favors paradoxical growth and cell survival. Breast Cancer Res. 2009;11(6):R81.

107. Siddiqui EJ, Shabbir MA, Mikhailidis DP, Mumtaz FH, Thompson CS. The effect of serotonin and serotonin antagonists on bladder cancer cell proliferation. BJU Int. 2006;97(3):634-9.

108. Sui H, Xu H, Ji Q, et al. 5-hydroxytryptamine receptor (5-HT1DR) promotes colorectal cancer metastasis by regulating Axin1/β-catenin/MMP-7 signaling pathway. Oncotarget. 2015;6(28):25975-87.

109. Koh KJ, Pearce AL, Marshman G, Finlay-jones JJ, Hart PH. Tea tree oil reduces histamine-induced skin inflammation. Br J Dermatol. 2002;147(6):1212-7.

110. Adlesic M, Verdrengh M, Bokarewa M, Dahlberg L, Foster SJ, Tarkowski A. Histamine in rheumatoid arthritis. Scand J Immunol. 2007;65(6):530-7.

111. Lefranc F, Yeaton P, Brotchi J, Kiss R. Cimetidine, an unexpected anti-tumor agent, and its potential for the treatment of glioblastoma (review). Int J Oncol. 2006;28(5):1021-30.

112. Hsieh HY, Shen CH, Lin RI, et al. Cyproheptadine exhibits antitumor activity in urothelial carcinoma cells by targeting GSK3β to suppress mTOR and β-catenin signaling pathways. Cancer Lett. 2016;370(1):56-65.

113. Harris AL, Smith IE. Regression of carcinoid tumour with cyproheptadine. Br Med J (Clin Res Ed). 1982;285(6340):475.

114. Choi SY, Collins CC, Gout PW, Wang Y. Cancer-generated lactic acid: a regulatory, immunosuppressive metabolite?. J Pathol. 2013;230(4):350-5.

115. Dhup S, Dadhich RK, Porporato PE, Sonveaux P. Multiple biological activities of lactic acid in cancer: influences on tumor growth, angiogenesis and metastasis. Curr Pharm Des. 2012;18(10):1319-30.

116. Wahl P, Zinner C, Achtzehn S, Bloch W, Mester J. Effect of high- and low-intensity exercise and metabolic acidosis on levels of GH, IGF-I, IGFBP-3 and cortisol. Growth Horm IGF Res. 2010;20(5):380-5.

117. Brand JM, Frohn C, Cziupka K, Brockmann C, Kirchner H, Luhm J. Prolactin triggers pro-inflammatory immune responses in peripheral immune cells. Eur Cytokine Netw. 2004;15(2):99-104.

118. Tworoger SS, Eliassen AH, Zhang X, et al. A 20-year prospective study of plasma prolactin as a risk marker of breast cancer development. Cancer Res. 2013;73(15):4810-9.

119. Clevenger, C.V. Role of Prolactin/Prolactin Receptor Signaling in Human Breast Cancer. Breast Disease. 18(1):75.

120. Recchione C, Galante E, Secreto G, Cavalleri A, Dati V. Abnormal serum hormone levels in lung cancer. Tumori. 1983;69(4):293-8.

121. Capuron L, Ravaud A, Neveu PJ, Miller AH, Maes M, Dantzer R. Association between decreased serum tryptophan concentrations and depressive symptoms in cancer patients undergoing cytokine therapy. Mol Psychiatry. 2002;7(5):468-73.

122. Håkanson E, Rutberg H, Jorfeldt L. Effect of adrenaline on exchange of free fatty acids in leg tissues and splanchnic area. A comparison with the metabolic

response to surgical stress. Clin Physiol. 1986;6(5):453-63.

123. Coppack SW, Jensen MD, Miles JM. In vivo regulation of lipolysis in humans. J Lipid Res. 1994;35(2):177-93.

124. Lee CG, Link H, Baluk P, et al. Vascular endothelial growth factor (VEGF) induces remodeling and enhances TH2-mediated sensitization and inflammation in the lung. Nat Med. 2004;10(10):1095-103.

125. Manzoor H, Qadir MI, Abbas K, et al. Vascular endothelial growth factor (VEGF) in cancer. African journal of pharmacy and pharmacology. 2014;8(37):917-923.

126. Sasaki T, Hiroki K, Yamashita Y. The role of epidermal growth factor receptor in cancer metastasis and microenvironment. Biomed Res Int. 2013;2013:546318.

127. Koenders PG, Beex LV, Kienhuis CB, Kloppenborg PW, Benraad TJ. Epidermal growth factor receptor and prognosis in human breast cancer: a prospective study. Breast Cancer Res Treat. 1993;25(1):21-7.

128. Waldner MJ, Foersch S, Neurath MF. Interleukin-6--a key regulator of colorectal cancer development. Int J Biol Sci. 2012;8(9):1248-53.

129. Lentz EK, Cherla RP, Jaspers V, Weeks BR, Tesh VL. Role of tumor necrosis factor alpha in disease using a mouse model of Shiga toxin-mediated renal damage. Infect Immun. 2010;78(9):3689-99.

130. Mocellin S, Rossi CR, Pilati P, Nitti D. Tumor necrosis factor, cancer and anticancer therapy. Cytokine Growth Factor Rev. 2005;16(1):35-53.

131. Ulich TR, Del castillo J, Ni RX, Bikhazi N, Calvin L. Mechanisms of tumor necrosis factor alpha-induced lymphopenia, neutropenia, and biphasic neutrophilia: a study of lymphocyte recirculation and hematologic interactions of TNF alpha with endogenous mediators of leukocyte trafficking. J Leukoc Biol. 1989;45(2):155-67.

132. Clark GC, Taylor MJ. Tumor necrosis factor involvement in the toxicity of TCDD: the role of endotoxin in the response. Exp Clin Immunogenet. 1994;11(2-3):136-41.

133. Degasperi GR, Romanatto T, Denis RG, et al. UCP2 protects hypothalamic cells from TNF-alpha-induced damage. FEBS Lett. 2008;582(20):3103-10.

134. Han D, Hosokawa T, Aoike A, Kawai K. Age-related enhancement of tumor necrosis factor (TNF) production in mice. Mech Ageing Dev. 1995;84(1):39-54.

135. Schmidlin K, Spoerri A, Egger M, et al. Cancer, a disease of aging (part 1) - trends in older adult cancer mortality in Switzerland 1991-2008. Swiss Med Wkly. 2012;142:w13637.

136. Pinna F, Sahle S, Beuke K, et al. A Systems Biology Study on NFκB Signaling in Primary Mouse Hepatocytes. Front Physiol. 2012;3:466.

137. Wang S, Liu Z, Wang L, Zhang X. NF-kappaB signaling pathway, inflammation and colorectal cancer. Cell Mol Immunol. 2009;6(5):327-34.

138. Sakamoto K, Maeda S, Hikiba Y, et al. Constitutive NF-kappaB activation in colorectal carcinoma plays a key role in angiogenesis, promoting tumor growth. Clin Cancer Res. 2009;15(7):2248-58.

139. Bharti AC, Aggarwal BB. Nuclear factor-kappa B and cancer: its role in prevention and therapy. Biochem Pharmacol. 2002;64(5-6):883-8.

140. Olivier S, Robe P, Bours V. Can NF-kappaB be a target for novel and efficient anti-cancer agents?. Biochem Pharmacol. 2006;72(9):1054-68.

141. Weber J, Yang JC, Topalian SL, et al. Phase I trial of subcutaneous interleukin-6 in patients with advanced malignancies. J Clin Oncol. 1993;11(3):499-506.

142. Weiss GR, Margolin KA, Sznol M, et al. A phase II study of the continuous intravenous infusion of interleukin-6 for metastatic renal cell carcinoma. J Immunother Emphasis Tumor Immunol. 1995;18(1):52-6

143. Shalowitz DI, Epstein AJ, Buckingham L, Ko EM, Giuntoli RL. Survival implications of time to surgical treatment of endometrial cancers. Am J Obstet Gynecol. 2016.

144. Bethune R, Sbaih M, Brosnan C, Arulampalam T. What happens when we do not operate? Survival following conservative bowel cancer management. Ann R Coll Surg Engl. 2016;98(6):409-12.

145. Tang D, Kang R, Zeh HJ, Lotze MT. High-mobility group box 1 and cancer. Biochim Biophys Acta. 2010;1799(1-2):131-40.

146. Okada S, Okusaka T, Ishii H, et al. Elevated serum interleukin-6 levels in patients with pancreatic cancer. Jpn J Clin Oncol. 1998;28(1):12-5.

147. Tian G, Mi J, Wei X, et al. Circulating interleukin-6 and cancer: A meta-analysis using Mendelian randomization. Sci Rep. 2015;5:11394.

148. Lobo V, Patil A, Phatak A, Chandra N. Free radicals, antioxidants and functional foods: Impact on human health. Pharmacogn Rev. 2010;4(8):118-26.

149. Chen Q, Guan X, Zuo X, Wang J, Yin W. The role of high mobility group box 1 (HMGB1) in the pathogenesis of kidney diseases. Acta Pharm Sin B. 2016;6(3):183-8.

CHEMOTHERAPY

1. (2014). Evolution of Cancer Treatments: Chemotherapy. [Online] Available: http://www.cancer.org/cancer/cancerbasics/thchistoryofcancer/the-history-of-cancer-cancer-treatment-chemo. [November 28, 2016].

2. Dickerson, C. (2015). *Families React To NPR's Reporting Of Secret Mustard Gas Testing.* [Online]. Available: http://www.npr.org/2015/11/03/453962074/familics-react-to-nprs-reporting-of-secret-mustard-gas-testing. [November 28, 2016].

3. (2011). Chemical Weapons Specialist Helps WWII Veteran Find Effective Treatment For Mustard Gas Symptoms. [Online]. Available: http://www.cdc.gov/nceh/stories/mustard_gas.html. [November 28, 2016].

4. Gilman A. Therapeutic applications of chemical warfare agents. Fed Proc. 1946;5:285-92.

5. Goodman LS, Wintrobe MM. Nitrogen mustard therapy; use of methyl-bis (beta-chloroethyl) amine hydrochloride and tris (beta-chloroethyl) amine hydrochloride for Hodgkin's disease, lymphosarcoma, leukemia and certain allied and miscellaneous disorders. J Am Med Assoc. 1946;132:126-32.

6. Gilman A, Philips FS. The Biological Actions and Therapeutic Applications of the B-Chloroethyl Amines and Sulfides. Science. 1946;103(2675):409-36.

7. The Gerson Institute. *Dr. Gerson's Suppressed 1946 Congressional Testimony.* [Online]. Available: http://whale.to/cancer/dr_gerson.html. [November 28, 2016].

8. iHealthTube.com, Gonzales, N. (2012). *The Shocking History of Chemotherapy.* [YouTube]. Available: https://www.youtube.com/watch?v=_TptKbxQJr4. [November 28, 2016].

9. Powles TJ, Coombes RC, Smith IE, Jones JM, Ford HT, Gazet JC. Failure of chemotherapy to prolong survival in a group of patients with metastatic breast cancer. Lancet. 1980;1(8168 Pt 1):580-2.

10. Blech, Jorg. (2004). *Giftkur ohne Nutzen.* [Online]. Available: http://www.spiegel.de/spiegel/print/d-32362278.html [November 28, 2016].

11. Abel, Ulrich, PhD "Cytostatic Therapy of Advanced Epithelial Tumors – A Critique" Lancet 10 Aug 1991.

12. Morgan G, Ward R, Barton M. The contribution of cytotoxic chemotherapy to 5-year survival in adult

malignancies. Clin Oncol (R Coll Radiol). 2004;16(8):549-60.

13. Markstein M, Dettorre S, Cho J, Neumüller RA, Craig-müller S, Perrimon N. Systematic screen of chemotherapeutics in Drosophila stem cell tumors. Proc Natl Acad Sci USA. 2014;111(12):4530-5.

14. Wallington M, Saxon EB, Bomb M, et al. 30-day mortality after systemic anticancer treatment for breast and lung cancer in England: a population-based, observational study. Lancet Oncol. 2016;17(9):1203-16.

15. Owusu C, Margevicius S, Schluchter M, Koroukian SM, Schmitz KH, Berger NA. Vulnerable elders survey and socioeconomic status predict functional decline and death among older women with newly diagnosed nonmetastatic breast cancer. Cancer. 2016;122(16):2579-86.

16. Bayraktar S, Garcia-buitrago MT, Hurley E, Gluck S. Surviving metastatic breast cancer for 18 years: a case report and review of the literature. Breast J. 2011;17(5):521-4.

17. Fernandes NM, Pelissari IG, Cogo LA, Santos filha VA. Workplace Activity in Health Professionals Exposed to Chemotherapy Drugs: An Otoneurological Perspective. Int Arch Otorhinolaryngol. 2016;20(4):331-338.

18. Drugs.com. (2013). *Mustargen.* [Online]. Available: https://www.drugs.com/pro/mustargen.html [November 28, 2016].

19. Mountzios G, Aravantinos G, Alexopoulou Z, et al. Lessons from the past: Long-term safety and survival

outcomes of a prematurely terminated randomized controlled trial on prophylactic vs. hemoglobin-based administration of erythropoiesis-stimulating agents in patients with chemotherapy-induced anemia. Mol Clin Oncol. 2016;4(2):211-220.

20. Li DY, Yu TT, Bai H, Chen XY. [Clinical study on effect of compound granule prescription of thunberg fritillary bulb in relieving post-chemotherapy bone marrow suppression in RAL patients]. Zhongguo Zhong Yao Za Zhi. 2012;37(20):3155-7.

21. Tamamyan G, Danielyan S, Lambert MP. Chemotherapy induced thrombocytopenia in pediatric oncology. Crit Rev Oncol Hematol. 2016;99:299-307.

22. Antonuzzo L, Lunghi A, Giommoni E, Brugia M, Di costanzo F. Regorafenib Also Can Cause Osteonecrosis of the Jaw. J Natl Cancer Inst. 2016;108(4).

23. Bordbar MR, Haghpanah S, Dabbaghmanesh MH, Omrani GR, Saki F. Bone mineral density in children with acute leukemia and its associated factors in Iran: a case-control study. Arch Osteoporos. 2016;11(1):36.

24. Lee SW, Yeo SG, Oh IH, Yeo JH, Park DC. Bone mineral density in women treated for various types of gynecological cancer. Asia Pac J Clin Oncol. 2016;

25. Matsuoka A, Mitsuma A, Maeda O, et al. Quantitative assessment of chemotherapy-induced peripheral neurotoxicity using a point-of-care nerve conduction device. Cancer Sci. 2016;107(10):1453-1457.

26. Iarkov A, Appunn D, Echeverria V. Post-treatment with cotinine improved memory and decreased

depressive-like behavior after chemotherapy in rats. Cancer Chemother Pharmacol. 2016;78(5):1033-1039.

27. Rendeiro C, Sheriff A, Bhattacharya TK, et al. Long-lasting impairments in adult neurogenesis, spatial learning and memory from a standard chemotherapy regimen used to treat breast cancer. Behav Brain Res. 2016;315:10-22.

28. Reddy AT, Witek K. Neurologic complications of chemotherapy for children with cancer. Curr Neurol Neurosci Rep. 2003;3(2):137-42.

29. Dunn J, Watson M, Aitken JF, Hyde MK. Systematic Review of Psychosocial Outcomes for Patients with Advanced Melanoma. Psychooncology. 2016;

30. Oh PJ, Lee JR. [Effect of Cancer Symptoms and Fatigue on Chemotherapy-related Cognitive Impairment and Depression in People with Gastrointestinal Cancer]. J Korean Acad Nurs. 2016;46(3):420-30.

31. Baek Y, Yi M. [Factors Influencing Quality of Life during Chemotherapy for Colorectal Cancer Patients in South Korea]. J Korean Acad Nurs. 2015;45(4):604-12.

32. Peretz B, Sarnat H, Kharouba J. Chemotherapy induced dental changes in a child with medulloblastoma: a case report. J Clin Pediatr Dent. 2014;38(3):251-4.

33. Alt-epping B, Nejad RK, Jung K, Gross U, Nauck F. Symptoms of the oral cavity and their association with local microbiological and clinical findings--a prospective survey in palliative care. Support Care Cancer. 2012;20(3):531-7.

34. Dreizen S, Mccredie KB, Keating MJ. Chemotherapy-induced oral mucositis in adult leukemia. Postgrad Med. 1981;69(2):103-8, 111-2.

35. Farsi DJ. Children Undergoing Chemotherapy: Is It Too Late for Dental Rehabilitation?. J Clin Pediatr Dent. 2016;40(6):503-505.

36. Abalo R, Uranga JA, Pérez-garcía I, et al. May cannabinoids prevent the development of chemotherapy-induced diarrhea and intestinal mucositis? Experimental study in the rat. Neurogastroenterol Motil. 2016.

37. Forsgård RA, Korpela R, Holma R, et al. Intestinal permeability to iohexol as an in vivo marker of chemotherapy-induced gastrointestinal toxicity in Sprague-Dawley rats. Cancer Chemother Pharmacol. 2016;78(4):863-74.

38. Klepin HD, Tooze JA, Pardee TS, et al. Effect of Intensive Chemotherapy on Physical, Cognitive, and Emotional Health of Older Adults with Acute Myeloid Leukemia. J Am Geriatr Soc. 2016;64(10):1988-1995.

39. Gilliam LA, Lark DS, Reese LR, et al. Targeted overexpression of mitochondrial catalase protects against cancer chemotherapy-induced skeletal muscle dysfunction. Am J Physiol Endocrinol Metab. 2016;311(2):E293-301.

40. Giralt J, Rey A, Villanueva R, Alforja S, Casaroli-marano RP. Severe visual loss in a breast cancer patient on chemotherapy. Med Oncol. 2012;29(4):2567-9.

41. Cloutier AO. Ocular side effects of chemotherapy: nursing management. Oncol Nurs Forum. 1992;19(8):1251-9.

42. Batchvarov IS, Taylor RW, Bustamante-marín X, et al. A grafted ovarian fragment rescues host fertility after chemotherapy. Mol Hum Reprod. 2016.

43. Clowse ME, Behera MA, Anders CK, et al. Ovarian preservation by GnRH agonists during chemotherapy: a meta-analysis. J Womens Health (Larchmt). 2009;18(3):311-9.

44. Garrido-oyarzún MF, Castelo-branco C. Controversies over the use of GnRH agonists for reduction of chemotherapy-induced gonadotoxicity. Climacteric. 2016;19(6):522-525.

45. Li CY, Chen ML. [Chemotherapy-Induced Amenorrhea and Menopause Symptoms in Women With Breast Cancer]. Hu Li Za Zhi. 2016;63(5):19-26.

46. Eid AH, Abdelkader NF, Abd el-raouf OM, Fawzy HM, El-denshary ES. Carvedilol alleviates testicular and spermatological damage induced by cisplatin in rats via modulation of oxidative stress and inflammation. Arch Pharm Res. 2016.

47. Levi M, Popovtzer A, Tzabari M, et al. Cetuximab intensifies cisplatin-induced testicular toxicity. Reprod Biomed Online. 2016;33(1):102-10.

48. Huang M, Lin J, Yu X, et al. Erectile and urinary function in men with rectal cancer treated by neoadjuvant chemoradiotherapy and neoadjuvant chemotherapy alone: a randomized trial report. Int J Colorectal Dis. 2016;31(7):1349-57.

49. Annam K, Voznesensky M, Kreder KJ. Understanding and Managing Erectile Dysfunction in Patients Treated for Cancer. J Oncol Pract. 2016;12(4):297-304.

50. Trüeb RM. Chemotherapy-induced alopecia. Semin Cutan Med Surg. 2009;28(1):11-4.

51. Tanaka S, Hayek G, Jayapratap P, et al. The Impact of Chemotherapy on Complications Associated with Mastectomy and Immediate Autologous Tissue Reconstruction. Am Surg. 2016;82(8):713-7.

52. Frisina RD, Wheeler HE, Fossa SD, et al. Comprehensive Audiometric Analysis of Hearing Impairment and Tinnitus After Cisplatin-Based Chemotherapy in Survivors of Adult-Onset Cancer. J Clin Oncol. 2016;34(23):2712-20.

53. Truong J, Yan AT, Cramarossa G, Chan KK. Chemotherapy-induced cardiotoxicity: detection, prevention, and management. Can J Cardiol. 2014;30(8):869-78.

54. Granger CB. Prediction and prevention of chemotherapy-induced cardiomyopathy: can it be done?. Circulation. 2006;114(23):2432-3.

55. Smith SA, Auseon AJ. Chemotherapy-induced takotsubo cardiomyopathy. Heart Fail Clin. 2013;9(2):233-42.

56. Sakka S, Kawai K, Tsujimoto I, et al. [Severe Acute Myocardial Infarction during Induction Chemotherapy for Retroperitoneal Germ Cell Tumor : A Case Report]. Hinyokika Kiyo. 2016;62(9):483-487.

57. Perkins JL, Harris A, Pozos TC. Immune Dysfunction After Completion of Childhood Leukemia Therapy. J Pediatr Hematol Oncol. 2016.

58. Verma R, Foster RE, Horgan K, et al. Lymphocyte depletion and repopulation after chemotherapy for primary breast cancer. Breast Cancer Res. 2016;18(1):10.

59. Lin JW, Chang ML, Hsu CW, et al. Acute exacerbation of hepatitis C in hepatocellular carcinoma patients receiving chemotherapy. J Med Virol. 2017;89(1):153-160.

60. Qin L, Wang F, Zou BW, Ding ZY. Chemotherapy-induced fatal hepatitis B virus reactivation in a small cell lung cancer patient. Mol Clin Oncol. 2016;5(4):382-384.

61. Wu Y, Deng Z, Wang H, Ma W, Zhou C, Zhang S. Repeated cycles of 5-fluorouracil chemotherapy impaired anti-tumor functions of cytotoxic T cells in a CT26 tumor-bearing mouse model. BMC Immunol. 2016;17(1):29.

62. Li W, Yan MH, Liu Y, et al. Ginsenoside Rg5 Ameliorates Cisplatin-Induced Nephrotoxicity in Mice through Inhibition of Inflammation, Oxidative Stress, and Apoptosis. Nutrients. 2016;8(9).

63. El-naga RN. Pre-treatment with cardamonin protects against cisplatin-induced nephrotoxicity in rats: impact on NOX-1, inflammation and apoptosis. Toxicol Appl Pharmacol. 2014;274(1):87-95.

64. Tiong V, Rozita AM, Taib NA, Yip CH, Ng CH. Incidence of chemotherapy-induced ovarian failure in

premenopausal women undergoing chemotherapy for breast cancer. World J Surg. 2014;38(9):2288-96.

65. Dugbartey GJ, Peppone LJ, De graaf IA. An integrative view of cisplatin-induced renal and cardiac toxicities: Molecular mechanisms, current treatment challenges and potential protective measures. Toxicology. 2016;371:58-66.

66. Hiroshima Y, Shuto K, Yamazaki K, et al. Fractal Dimension of Tc-99m DTPA GSA Estimates Pathologic Liver Injury due to Chemotherapy in Liver Cancer Patients. Ann Surg Oncol. 2016;23(13):4384-4391.

67. Limper AH. Chemotherapy-induced lung disease. Clin Chest Med. 2004;25(1):53-64.

68. Berger velten D, Zandonade E, Monteiro de barros miotto MH. Prevalence of oral manifestations in children and adolescents with cancer submitted to chemotherapy. BMC Oral Health. 2016;16(1):107.

69. Gong SS, Li YX, Zhang MT, et al. Neuroprotective Effect of Matrine in Mouse Model of Vincristine-Induced Neuropathic Pain. Neurochem Res. 2016;41(11):3147-3159.

70. Hellerstedt-börjesson S, Nordin K, Fjällskog ML, Holmström IK, Arving C. Women Treated for Breast Cancer Experiences of Chemotherapy-Induced Pain: Memories, Any Present Pain, and Future Reflections. Cancer Nurs. 2016;39(6):464-472.

71. Mcnamara MJ, Adelstein DJ, Allende DS, et al. Persistent Dysphagia After Induction Chemotherapy in Patients with Esophageal Adenocarcinoma Predicts

Poor Post-Operative Outcomes. J Gastrointest Cancer. 2016.

72. Fakhfouri G, Mousavizadeh K, Mehr SE, et al. From Chemotherapy-Induced Emesis to Neuroprotection: Therapeutic Opportunities for 5-HT3 Receptor Antagonists. Mol Neurobiol. 2015;52(3):1670-9.

73. Thamlikitkul L, Srimuninnimit V, Akewanlop C, et al. Efficacy of ginger for prophylaxis of chemotherapy-induced nausea and vomiting in breast cancer patients receiving adriamycin-cyclophosphamide regimen: a randomized, double-blind, placebo-controlled, crossover study. Support Care Cancer. 2016.

74. Sozeri E, Kutluturkan S. The Validity and Reliability of Turkish Version of the Chemotherapy-induced Taste Alteration Scale (CiTAS). Clin Nurs Res. 2016.

75. Rajasekhar A, George TJ. Gemcitabine-induced reversible posterior leukoencephalopathy syndrome: a case report and review of the literature. Oncologist. 2007;12(11):1332-5.

76. Esquirol caussa J, Herrero vila E. [Epidermal growth factor, innovation and safety]. Med Clin (Barc). 2015;145(7):305-12.

77. Bagheri-nesami M, Goudarzian AH, Jan babaei G, Badiee M, Mousavi M, Sadegh sharifi M. Sleep Quality and Associated Risk Factors in Leukemia Patients Undergoing Chemotherapy in Iran. Asian Pac J Cancer Prev. 2016;17 Spec No.:107-11.

78. De groot S, Janssen LG, Charehbili A, et al. Thyroid function alters during neoadjuvant chemotherapy in breast cancer patients: results from the NEOZOTAC

trial (BOOG 2010-01). Breast Cancer Res Treat. 2015;149(2):461-6.

79. Anker GB, Lønning PE, Aakvaag A, Lien EA. Thyroid function in postmenopausal breast cancer patients treated with tamoxifen. Scand J Clin Lab Invest. 1998;58(2):103-7.

80. Khan MA, Bhurani D, Agarwal NB. Alteration of Thyroid Function in Indian HER 2-Negative Breast Cancer Patients Undergoing Chemotherapy. Asian Pac J Cancer Prev. 2015;16(17):7701-5.

81. Degener S, Pohle A, Strelow H, et al. Long-term experience of hyperbaric oxygen therapy for refractory radio- or chemotherapy-induced haemorrhagic cystitis. BMC Urol. 2015;15:38.

82. Nissinen TA, Degerman J, Räsänen M, et al. Systemic blockade of ACVR2B ligands prevents chemotherapy-induced muscle wasting by restoring muscle protein synthesis without affecting oxidative capacity or atrogenes. Sci Rep. 2016;6:32695.

83. Klose R, Krzywinska E, Castells M, et al. Targeting VEGF-A in myeloid cells enhances natural killer cell responses to chemotherapy and ameliorates cachexia. Nat Commun. 2016;7:12528.

84. Mukaida K, Hattori N, Iwamoto H, et al. Mustard gas exposure and mortality among retired workers at a poisonous gas factory in Japan: a 57-year follow-up cohort study. Occup Environ Med. 2016.

85. Limberaki E, Eleftheriou P, Gasparis G, Karalekos E, Kostoglou V, Petrou C. Cortisol levels and serum antioxidant status following chemotherapy. 2012; Available at:

https://www.researchgate.net/publication/224943223
_Cortisol_levels_and_serum_antioxidant_status_follo
wing_chemotherapy. [December 1, 2016].

86. Lalla RV, Pilbeam CC, Walsh SJ, Sonis ST, Keefe DM, Peterson DE. Role of the cyclooxygenase pathway in chemotherapy-induced oral mucositis: a pilot study. Support Care Cancer. 2010;18(1):95-103.

87. Kondo K, Fujiwara M, Murase M, et al. Severe acute metabolic acidosis and Wernicke's encephalopathy following chemotherapy with 5-fluorouracil and cisplatin: case report and review of the literature. Jpn J Clin Oncol. 1996;26(4):234-6.

88. Cubeddu LX, Hoffmann IS, Fuenmayor NT, Malave JJ. Changes in serotonin metabolism in cancer patients: its relationship to nausea and vomiting induced by chemotherapeutic drugs. Br J Cancer. 1992;66(1):198-203.

89. Eschalier A, Lavarenne J, Burtin C, Renoux M, Chapuy E, Rodriguez M. Study of histamine release induced by acute administration of antitumor agents in dogs. Cancer Chemother Pharmacol. 1988;21(3):246-50.

90. Nguyen A, Bhavsar S, Riley E, Caponetti G, Agrawal D. Clinical Value of High Mobility Group Box 1 and the Receptor for Advanced Glycation End-products in Head and Neck Cancer: A Systematic Review. Int Arch Otorhinolaryngol. 2016;20(4):382-389.

91. Cheung YT, Ng T, Shwe M, et al. Association of proinflammatory cytokines and chemotherapy-associated cognitive impairment in breast cancer

patients: a multi-centered, prospective, cohort study. Ann Oncol. 2015;26(7):1446-51.

92. Waugh DJ, Wilson C. The interleukin-8 pathway in cancer. Clin Cancer Res. 2008;14(21):6735-41.

93. Tiligada E. Chemotherapy: induction of stress responses. Endocr Relat Cancer. 2006;13 Suppl 1(Supplement 1):S115-24.

94. Hinterberger-fischer M, Ogris E, Kier P, et al. Elevation of plasma prolactin in patients undergoing autologous blood stem-cell transplantation for breast cancer: is its modulation a step toward posttransplant immunotherapy?. Am J Clin Oncol. 2000;23(4):325-9.

95. Fan F, Gray MJ, Dallas NA, et al. Effect of chemotherapeutic stress on induction of vascular endothelial growth factor family members and receptors in human colorectal cancer cells. Mol Cancer Ther. 2008;7(9):3064-70.

96. Wang F, Liu R, Lee SW, Sloss CM, Couget J, Cusack JC. Heparin-binding EGF-like growth factor is an early response gene to chemotherapy and contributes to chemotherapy resistance. Oncogene. 2007;26(14):2006-16.

RADIOTHERAPY

1. Hall S, Rudrawar S, Zunk M, et al. Protection against Radiotherapy-Induced Toxicity. Antioxidants (Basel). 2016;5(3).

2. Nobel Lectures, *Physics 1901-1921*, Elsevier Publishing Company, Amsterdam, 1967. Available:

http://www.nobelprize.org/nobel_prizes/physics/laureates/1901/rontgen-bio.html.(December 1, 2016).

3. Moss, Ralph W. The cancer industry: the classic exposé on the cancer establishment. Brooklyn, NY: Equinox Press, 1996. Page 64.

4. Inglis-Arkell, E. (2011). *When X-rays were Given in Shoe Stores.* Gizmodo [Online]. Available: http://io9.gizmodo.com/5843183/when-x-rays-were-given-in-shoe-stores [February 24, 2016].

5. Smullen MJ, Bertler DE. Basal cell carcinoma of the sole: possible association with the shoe-fitting fluoroscope. WMJ. 2007;106(5):275-8.

6. Gofman, J. Lecture. Stinson Beach, California. 1999. *Medical X-rays and Breast Cancer.* Available: https://www.youtube.com/watch?v=AzW0zIjKcmE [February 24, 2016].

7. Peat, R. Audio Interview. 2009. *Radiation 2. Politics and Science.* Available: https://www.youtube.com/watch?v=7NjCopysMzo [February 24, 2016].

8. Yablokov AV, Nesterenko VB, Nesterenko AV et al. Chernobyl, Consequences of the Catastrophe for People and the Environment. John Wiley & Sons; 2010.

9. Allison, W. (2009). *Public Trust in Nuclear Energy.* [Online]. Available: http://docplayer.net/21237548-Public-trust-in-nuclear-energy.html. [December 1, 2016].

10. Adair, FE. (1943). The Role of Surgery and Irradiation in Cancer of The Breast. *JAMA.* 1943;121(8):553-559.

REFERENCES

11. Guttmann R. Radiotherapy in the treatment of primary operable carcinoma of the breast with proved lymph node metastases: approach and results. Am J Roentgenol Radium Ther Nucl Med. 1963;89:58-63.

12. Harrington SW. Results of surgical treatment of unilateral carcinoma of breast in women. J Am Med Assoc. 1952;148(12):1007-11.

13. Marshall SF, Hare HF. Carcinoma of the breast; results of combined treatment with surgery and roentgen rays. Ann Surg. 1947;125(6):688-702.

14. Watson TA. Carcinoma of the breast. Stage II-- radiation range. Can survival be increased by postoperative irradiation following radical mastectomy?. JAMA. 1967;200(2):136-7.

15. Butcher HR, Seaman WB, Eckert C, Saltzstein S. An Assessment Of Radical Mastectomy and Postoperative Irradiation Therapy In The Treatment Of Mammary Cancer. Cancer. 1964;17:480-5.

16. Cantrel, S. T. and Buschke, F.: The Role of Roentgen Therapy in Carcinoma of the Breast. West. J. Surg. Obstet. Gynec. 54: 369, 1946.

17. Chu FC, Lucas JC, Farrow JH, Nickson JJ. Does prophylactic radiation therapy given for cancer of the breast predispose to metastasis?. Am J Roentgenol Radium Ther Nucl Med. 1967;99(4):987-94.

18. Easson, E. C.: Postoperative Radiotherapy in Breast Cancer in Symposium on Prognostic Factors in Breast Cancer. (Edinburgh: Livingston, 1968), pp. 118-127.

19. Haagensen, C. D. and Stout, A. P.: Carcinoma of the Breast. I. Results of Treatment. Ann. Surg., 116:801, 1942.

20. Elkins HB, Hickey RC, Kerr HD, Tidrick RT, Wieben EE. Cancer of the breast, 1661 patients. I. Considerations in future therapy. AMA Arch Surg. 1956;73(4):654-60.

21. Paterson, Ralston, and Marion H. Russell. "Clinical Trials in Malignant Disease." *Journal of the Faculty of Radiologists* 10.4 (1959): 175–180.

22. Robbins GF, Lucas JC, Fracchia AA, Farrow JH, Chu FC. An evaluation of postoperative prophylactic radiation therapy in breast cancer. Surg Gynecol Obstet. 1966;122(5):979-82.

23. Treves N, Holleb AI. A report of 549 cases of breast cancer in women 35 years of age or younger. Surg Gynecol Obstet. 1958;107(3):271-83.

24. Dao, T. L. and Kovaric, J.: Incidence of Pulmonary and Skin Metastases in Women with Breast Cancer Who Received Postoperative Irradiation. Surgery, 52:203, 1962.

25. DeCourmelles, F.: Action Atrophique Glandulaire Des Rayons X. C. R. Acad. Sci (Paris), 140:606, 1905.

26. Fisher B, Slack NH, Cavanaugh PJ, Gardner B, Ravdin RG. Postoperative radiotherapy in the treatment of breast cancer: results of the NSABP clinical trial. Ann Surg. 1970;172(4):711-32.

27. Stjernswärd J. Decreased survival related to irradiation postoperatively in early operable breast cancer. Lancet. 1974;2(7892):1285-6.

28. Effects of radiotherapy and surgery in early breast cancer. An overview of the randomized trials. Early Breast Cancer Trialists' Collaborative Group. N Engl J Med. 1995;333(22):1444-55.

29. Postoperative radiotherapy in non-small-cell lung cancer: systematic review and meta-analysis of individual patient data from nine randomised controlled trials. PORT Meta-analysis Trialists Group. Lancet. 1998;352(9124):257-63.

30. Burdett S, Stewart L. Postoperative radiotherapy in non-small-cell lung cancer: update of an individual patient data meta-analysis. Lung Cancer. 2005;47(1):81-3.

31. Brown BW, Brauner C, Minnotte MC. Noncancer deaths in white adult cancer patients. J Natl Cancer Inst. 1993;85(12):979-87.

32. Adjuvant radiotherapy for rectal cancer: a systematic overview of 8,507 patients from 22 randomised trials. Lancet. 2001;358(9290):1291-304.

33. Clarke M, Collins R, Darby S, et al. Effects of radiotherapy and of differences in the extent of surgery for early breast cancer on local recurrence and 15-year survival: an overview of the randomised trials. Lancet. 2005;366(9503):2087-106.

34. Karadağ O, Demiröz abakay C, Özkan L, Sağlam H, Demirkaya M. Evaluation of late effects of postoperative radiotherapy in patients with medulloblastoma. Turk J Pediatr. 2015;57(2):167-71.

35. Kreiker J, Kattan J. Second colon cancer following Hodgkin's disease. A case report. J Med Liban. 1996;44(2):107-8.

36. Boulaâmane L, Tazi el M, Glaoui M, et al. [Hodgkin's disease and secondary colon cancer: report of a case]. Pan Afr Med J. 2011;9:25.

37. Kleinerman RA. Cancer risks following diagnostic and therapeutic radiation exposure in children. Pediatr Radiol. 2006;36 Suppl 2:121-5.

38. Shore RE, Moseson M, Xue X, Tse Y, Harley N, Pasternack BS. Skin cancer after X-ray treatment for scalp ringworm. Radiat Res. 2002;157(4):410-8.

39. Karagas MR, Nelson HH, Zens MS, et al. Squamous cell and basal cell carcinoma of the skin in relation to radiation therapy and potential modification of risk by sun exposure. Epidemiology. 2007;18(6):776-84.

40. Schellong G, Riepenhausen M, Ehlert K, et al. Breast cancer in young women after treatment for Hodgkin's disease during childhood or adolescence--an observational study with up to 33-year follow-up. Dtsch Arztebl Int. 2014;111(1-2):3-9.

41. Van den belt-dusebout AW, Aleman BM, Besseling G, et al. Roles of radiation dose and chemotherapy in the etiology of stomach cancer as a second malignancy. Int J Radiat Oncol Biol Phys. 2009;75(5):1420-9.

42. Hancock SL, Tucker MA, Hoppe RT. Breast cancer after treatment of Hodgkin's disease. J Natl Cancer Inst. 1993;85(1):25-31.

43. Hauptmann M, Børge johannesen T, Gilbert ES, et al. Increased pancreatic cancer risk following radiotherapy for testicular cancer. Br J Cancer. 2016;115(7):901-8.

44. Hauptmann M, Fossa SD, Stovall M, et al. Increased stomach cancer risk following radiotherapy for testicular cancer. Br J Cancer. 2015;112(1):44-51.

45. Griem ML, Kleinerman RA, Boice JD, Stovall M, Shefner D, Lubin JH. Cancer following radiotherapy for peptic ulcer. J Natl Cancer Inst. 1994;86(11):842-9.

46. Lawrence TS, Ten Haken RK, Giaccia A. Principles of Radiation Oncology. In: DeVita VT Jr., Lawrence TS, Rosenberg SA, editors. *Cancer: Principles and Practice of Oncology.* 8th ed. Philadelphia: Lippincott Williams and Wilkins, 2008.

47. Nagasawa H, Little JB. Induction of sister chromatid exchanges by extremely low doses of alpha-particles. Cancer Res. 1992;52(22):6394-6.

48. Koturbash I, Kutanzi K, Hendrickson K, Rodriguez-juarez R, Kogosov D, Kovalchuk O. Radiation-induced bystander effects in vivo are sex specific. Mutat Res. 2008;642(1-2):28-36.

49. Mothersill C, Bucking C, Smith RW, et al. Communication of radiation-induced stress or bystander signals between fish in vivo. Environ Sci Technol. 2006;40(21):6859-64.

50. Khan MA, Van dyk J, Yeung IW, Hill RP. Partial volume rat lung irradiation; assessment of early DNA damage in different lung regions and effect of radical scavengers. Radiother Oncol. 2003;66(1):95-102.

51. Kovalchuk A, Mychasiuk R, Muhammad A, et al. Liver irradiation causes distal bystander effects in the rat brain and affects animal behaviour. Oncotarget. 2016;7(4):4385-98.

52. Koturbash I, Loree J, Kutanzi K, Koganow C, Pogribny I, Kovalchuk O. In vivo bystander effect: cranial X-irradiation leads to elevated DNA damage, altered cellular proliferation and apoptosis, and increased p53 levels in shielded spleen. Int J Radiat Oncol Biol Phys. 2008;70(2):554-62.

53. Whiteside JR, Mcmillan TJ. A bystander effect is induced in human cells treated with UVA radiation but not UVB radiation. Radiat Res. 2009;171(2):204-11.

54. Hujoel PP, Bollen AM, Noonan CJ, Del aguila MA. Antepartum dental radiography and infant low birth weight. JAMA. 2004;291(16):1987-93.

55. Li F, Liu P, Wang T, et al. The induction of bystander mutagenic effects in vivo by alpha-particle irradiation in whole Arabidopsis thaliana plants. Radiat Res. 2010;174(2):228-37.

56. Shao C, Folkard M, Prise KM. Role of TGF-beta1 and nitric oxide in the bystander response of irradiated glioma cells. Oncogene. 2008;27(4):434-40.

57. Yakovlev VA. Role of nitric oxide in the radiation-induced bystander effect. Redox Biol. 2015;6:396-400.

58. Han W, Wu L, Chen S, et al. Constitutive nitric oxide acting as a possible intercellular signaling molecule in the initiation of radiation-induced DNA double strand breaks in non-irradiated bystander cells. Oncogene. 2007;26(16):2330-9.

59. Xiao L, Liu W, Li J, et al. Irradiated U937 cells trigger inflammatory bystander responses in human umbilical vein endothelial cells through the p38 pathway. Radiat Res. 2014;182(1):111-21.

60. Peer G, Itzhakov E, Wollman Y, et al. Methylene blue, a nitric oxide inhibitor, prevents haemodialysis hypotension. Nephrol Dial Transplant. 2001;16(7):1436-41.

61. Sokolov MV, Smilenov LB, Hall EJ, Panyutin IG, Bonner WM, Sedelnikova OA. Ionizing radiation induces DNA double-strand breaks in bystander primary human fibroblasts. Oncogene. 2005;24(49):7257-65.

62. Shao C, Folkard M, Held KD, Prise KM. Estrogen enhanced cell-cell signalling in breast cancer cells exposed to targeted irradiation. BMC Cancer. 2008;8:184.

63. Boroujerdi, A. Estrogen Exposure Rapidly Elevates Nitric Oxide Production in Cerebral Vessels. [Online]. Available: http://www.urop.uci.edu/journal/journal03/01_Ami nBoroujerdi/boroujerdi.pdf [December 1, 2016].

64. García-durán M, De frutos T, Díaz-recasens J, et al. Estrogen stimulates neuronal nitric oxide synthase protein expression in human neutrophils. Circ Res. 1999;85(11):1020-6.

65. Han W, Wu L, Chen S, et al. Constitutive nitric oxide acting as a possible intercellular signaling molecule in the initiation of radiation-induced DNA double strand breaks in non-irradiated bystander cells. Oncogene. 2007;26(16):2330-9.

66. Sypniewska RK, Millenbaugh NJ, Kiel JL, et al. Protein changes in macrophages induced by plasma from rats exposed to 35 GHz millimeter waves. Bioelectromagnetics. 2010;31(8):656-63.

67. Pall ML. Electromagnetic fields act via activation of voltage-gated calcium channels to produce beneficial or adverse effects. J Cell Mol Med. 2013;17(8):958-65.

68. Myung SK, Ju W, Mcdonnell DD, et al. Mobile phone use and risk of tumors: a meta-analysis. J Clin Oncol. 2009;27(33):5565-72.

69. Hardell L, Carlberg M, Söderqvist F, Mild KH. Case-control study of the association between malignant brain tumours diagnosed between 2007 and 2009 and mobile and cordless phone use. Int J Oncol. 2013;43(6):1833-45.

70. Morgan LL, Miller AB, Sasco A, Davis DL. Mobile phone radiation causes brain tumors and should be classified as a probable human carcinogen (2A) (review). Int J Oncol. 2015;46(5):1865-71.

71. Crocetti E, Trama A, Stiller C, et al. Epidemiology of glial and non-glial brain tumours in Europe. Eur J Cancer. 2012;48(10):1532-42.

72. Coureau G, Bouvier G, Lebailly P, et al. Mobile phone use and brain tumours in the CERENAT case-control study. Occup Environ Med. 2014;71(7):514-22.

73. Benson VS, Pirie K, Schüz J, et al. Mobile phone use and risk of brain neoplasms and other cancers: prospective study. Int J Epidemiol. 2013;42(3):792-802.

74. Sadetzki S, Chetrit A, Jarus-hakak A, et al. Cellular phone use and risk of benign and malignant parotid gland tumors--a nationwide case-control study. Am J Epidemiol. 2008;167(4):457-67.

75. Karipidis KK, Benke G, Sim MR, et al. Occupational exposure to ionizing and non-ionizing radiation and risk of non-Hodgkin lymphoma. Int Arch Occup Environ Health. 2007;80(8):663-70.

76. West JG, Kapoor NS, Liao SY, Chen JW, Bailey L, Nagourney RA. Multifocal Breast Cancer in Young Women with Prolonged Contact between Their Breasts and Their Cellular Phones. Case Rep Med. 2013;2013:354682.

77. Stang A, Anastassiou G, Ahrens W, Bromen K, Bornfeld N, Jöckel KH. The possible role of radiofrequency radiation in the development of uveal melanoma. Epidemiology. 2001;12(1):7-12.

78. Lala PK, Chakraborty C. Role of nitric oxide in carcinogenesis and tumour progression. Lancet Oncol. 2001;2(3):149-56.

79. Engin AB. Dual function of nitric oxide in carcinogenesis, reappraisal. Curr Drug Metab. 2011;12(9):891-9.

80. Shimon I, Manisterski Y, Kanner AA. Acute cortisol release during stereotactic fractionated radiotherapy to an ACTH-secreting pituitary macroadenoma. Pituitary. 2012;15 Suppl 1:S41-5.

81. Sonveaux P, Brouet A, Havaux X, et al. Irradiation-induced angiogenesis through the up-regulation of the nitric oxide pathway: implications for tumor radiotherapy. Cancer Res. 2003;63(5):1012-9.

82. Hovinga KE, Stalpers LJ, Van bree C, et al. Radiation-enhanced vascular endothelial growth factor (VEGF) secretion in glioblastoma multiforme cell lines--a clue to radioresistance?. J Neurooncol. 2005;74(2):99-103.

83. Ozbilgin MK, Aktas C, Uluer ET, Buyukuysal MC, Gareveran MS, Kurtman C. Influence of Radiation Exposure During Radiotherapy. Evidence for the Increase of Versican and Heparin-Binding EGF-like Growth Factor Concentrations. Anal Quant Cytopathol Histpathol. 2016;38(2):126-32.

84. Kim ES, Choi YE, Hwang SJ, Han YH, Park MJ, Bae IH. IL-4, a direct target of miR-340/429, is involved in radiation-induced aggressive tumor behavior in human carcinoma cells. Oncotarget. 2016.

85. Tabatabaei P, Visse E, Bergström P, Brännström T, Siesjö P, Bergenheim AT. Radiotherapy induces an immediate inflammatory reaction in malignant glioma: a clinical microdialysis study. J Neurooncol. 2016.

86. Yeoh AS, Bowen JM, Gibson RJ, Keefe DM. Nuclear factor kappaB (NFkappaB) and cyclooxygenase-2 (Cox-2) expression in the irradiated colorectum is associated with subsequent histopathological changes. Int J Radiat Oncol Biol Phys. 2005;63(5):1295-303.

87. Ziboh VA, Mallia C, Morhart E, Taylor JR. Induced biosynthesis of cutaneous prostaglandins by ionizing irradiation. Proc Soc Exp Biol Med. 1982;169(3):386-91.

88. Ong ZY, Gibson RJ, Bowen JM, et al. Pro-inflammatory cytokines play a key role in the development of radiotherapy-induced gastrointestinal mucositis. Radiat Oncol. 2010;5:22.

89. Mccue JL, Sheffield JP, Phillips RK. Adjuvant radiotherapy and anastomosis in rectal cancer-- disturbing evidence from animal studies. Dis Colon Rectum. 1995;38(2):152-8.

90. Printz C. Radiation treatment generates therapy-resistant cancer stem cells from less aggressive breast cancer cells. Cancer. 2012;118(13):3225.

91. Whitcroft, I. (2008). Why won't our doctors face up to the dangers of radiotherapy? [Online]. Available: http://www.dailymail.co.uk/health/article-1089091/Why-wont-doctors-face-dangers-radiotherapy.html [December 1, 2016].

92. Bogdanich, W. (2010). Radiation Offers New Cures, and Ways to Do Harm. New York Times. [Online]. Available: http://www.nytimes.com/2010/01/24/health/24radiation.html [February 24, 2016].

93. Macbeth FR, Wheldon TE, Girling DJ, et al. Radiation myelopathy: estimates of risk in 1048 patients in three randomized trials of palliative radiotherapy for non-small cell lung cancer. The Medical Research Council Lung Cancer Working Party. Clin Oncol (R Coll Radiol). 1996;8(3):176-81.

94. Keus RB, Rutgers EJ, Ho GH, Gortzak E, Albus-lutter CE, Hart AA. Limb-sparing therapy of extremity soft tissue sarcomas: treatment outcome and long-term functional results. Eur J Cancer. 1994;30A(10):1459-63.

95. Hutchinson ID, Olson J, Lindburg CA, et al. Total-body irradiation produces late degenerative joint damage in rats. Int J Radiat Biol. 2014;90(9):821-30.

96. Kahalley LS, Ris MD, Grosshans DR, et al. Comparing Intelligence Quotient Change After Treatment With Proton Versus Photon Radiation Therapy for Pediatric Brain Tumors. J Clin Oncol. 2016;34(10):1043-9.

97. Greene-schloesser D, Robbins ME, Peiffer AM, Shaw EG, Wheeler KT, Chan MD. Radiation-induced brain injury: A review. Front Oncol. 2012;2:73.

98. Fernandez G, Pocinho R, Travancinha C, Netto E, Roldão M. Quality of life and radiotherapy in brain metastasis patients. Rep Pract Oncol Radiother. 2012;17(5):281-7.

99. Dorresteijn LD, Kappelle AC, Boogerd W, et al. Increased risk of ischemic stroke after radiotherapy on the neck in patients younger than 60 years. J Clin Oncol. 2002;20(1):282-8.

100. Uzun S, Toyran S, Akay F, Gundogan FC. Delayed visual loss due to radiation retinopathy. Pak J Med Sci. 2016;32(2):516-8.

101. Zeng KL, Kuruvilla S, Sanatani M, Louie AV. Bilateral Blindness Following Chemoradiation for Locally Advanced Oropharyngeal Carcinoma. Cureus. 2015;7(10):e352.

102. Metz JM, Smith D, Mick R, et al. A phase I study of topical Tempol for the prevention of alopecia induced by whole brain radiotherapy. Clin Cancer Res. 2004;10(19):6411-7.

103. Kiang JG, Garrison BR, Burns TM, et al. Wound trauma alters ionizing radiation dose assessment. Cell Biosci. 2012;2(1):20.

104. Wang Q, Dickson GR, Abram WP, Carr KE. Electron irradiation slows down wound repair in rat skin: a morphological investigation. Br J Dermatol. 1994;130(5):551-60.

105. Tibbs MK. Wound healing following radiation therapy: a review. Radiother Oncol. 1997;42(2):99-106.

106. Guimas V, Thariat J, Graff-cailleau P, et al. [Intensity modulated radiotherapy for head and neck cancer, dose constraint for normal tissue: Cochlea vestibular apparatus and brainstem]. Cancer Radiother. 2016;20(6-7):475-83.

107. Upadhya I, Jariwala N, Datar J. Ototoxic effects of irradiation. Indian J Otolaryngol Head Neck Surg. 2011;63(2):151-4.

108. Kirchmann M, Karnov K, Hansen S, Dethloff T, Stangerup SE, Caye-thomasen P. Ten-Year Follow-up on Tumor Growth and Hearing in Patients Observed With an Intracanalicular Vestibular Schwannoma. Neurosurgery. 2016.

109. Bass JK, Hua CH, Huang J, et al. Hearing Loss in Patients Who Received Cranial Radiation Therapy for Childhood Cancer. J Clin Oncol. 2016;34(11):1248-55.

110. Cuomo JR, Sharma GK, Conger PD, Weintraub NL. Novel concepts in radiation-induced cardiovascular disease. World J Cardiol. 2016;8(9):504-519.

111. Boivin JF, Hutchison GB, Lubin JH, Mauch P. Coronary artery disease mortality in patients treated for Hodgkin's disease. Cancer. 1992;69(5):1241-7.

112. Gyenes G, Rutqvist LE, Liedberg A, Fornander T. Long-term cardiac morbidity and mortality in a randomized trial of pre- and postoperative radiation therapy versus surgery alone in primary breast cancer. Radiother Oncol. 1998;48(2):185-90.

113. Fontanelli A, Bernardi G, Morocutti G, Di chiara A. [A case of radiation-induced coronary occlusion treated with elective and emergency PTCA]. G Ital Cardiol. 1995;25(7):877-84.

114. Roychoudhuri R, Robinson D, Putcha V, Cuzick J, Darby S, Møller H. Increased cardiovascular mortality more than fifteen years after radiotherapy for breast cancer: a population-based study. BMC Cancer. 2007;7:9.

115. Darby SC, Mcgale P, Taylor CW, Peto R. Long-term mortality from heart disease and lung cancer after radiotherapy for early breast cancer: prospective cohort study of about 300,000 women in US SEER cancer registries. Lancet Oncol. 2005;6(8):557-65.

116. Standish LJ, Torkelson C, Hamill FA, et al. Immune defects in breast cancer patients after radiotherapy. J Soc Integr Oncol. 2008;6(3):110-21.

117. Girod DA, Mcculloch TM, Tsue TT, Weymuller EA. Risk factors for complications in clean-contaminated head and neck surgical procedures. Head Neck. 1995;17(1):7-13.

118. Thorgersen EB, Goscinski MA, Spasojevic M, et al. Deep Pelvic Surgical Site Infection After Radiotherapy and Surgery for Locally Advanced Rectal Cancer. Ann Surg Oncol. 2016.

119. Lalla RV, Latortue MC, Hong CH, et al. A systematic review of oral fungal infections in patients receiving cancer therapy. Support Care Cancer. 2010;18(8):985-92.

120. Cheung JP, Mak KC, Tsang HH, Luk KD. A Lethal Sequelae of Spinal Infection Complicating Surgery and

Radiotherapy for Head and Neck Cancer. Asian Spine J. 2015;9(4):617-20.

121. Sbitany H, Wang F, Peled AW, et al. Immediate implant-based breast reconstruction following total skin-sparing mastectomy: defining the risk of preoperative and postoperative radiation therapy for surgical outcomes. Plast Reconstr Surg. 2014;134(3):396-404.

122. Low WK, Rangabashyam M, Wang F. Management of major post-cochlear implant wound infections. Eur Arch Otorhinolaryngol. 2014;271(9):2409-13.

123. De araujo TB, Jue xu M, Susarla SM, et al. Impact of Prior Unilateral Chest Wall Radiotherapy on Outcomes in Bilateral Breast Reconstruction. Plast Reconstr Surg. 2016;138(4):575-580.

124. Hughes MA, Parisi M, Grossman S, Kleinberg L. Primary brain tumors treated with steroids and radiotherapy: low CD4 counts and risk of infection. Int J Radiat Oncol Biol Phys. 2005;62(5):1423-6.

125. Azanan MS, Abdullah NK, Chua LL, et al. Immunity in young adult survivors of childhood leukemia is similar to the elderly rather than age-matched controls: Role of cytomegalovirus. Eur J Immunol. 2016;46(7):1715-26.

126. Tabatabaei P, Visse E, Bergström P, Brännström T, Siesjö P, Bergenheim AT. Radiotherapy induces an immediate inflammatory reaction in malignant glioma: a clinical microdialysis study. J Neurooncol. 2016.

127. Poskurica M, Petrović D, Poskurica M. [Acute renal failure in patients with tumour lysis sindrome]. Srp Arh Celok Lek. 2016;144(3-4):232-9.

128. Huang Y, Chen SW, Fan CC, Ting LL, Kuo CC, Chiou JF. Clinical parameters for predicting radiation-induced liver disease after intrahepatic reirradiation for hepatocellular carcinoma. Radiat Oncol. 2016;11(1):89.

129. Kitajima T, Fujimoto Y, Hatano E, et al. Salvage living-donor liver transplantation for liver failure following definitive radiation therapy for recurrent hepatocellular carcinoma: a case report. Transplant Proc. 2015;47(3):804-8.

130. Gebre-medhin M, Haghanegi M, Robért L, Kjellén E, Nilsson P. Dose-volume analysis of radiation-induced trismus in head and neck cancer patients. Acta Oncol. 2016;55(11):1313-1317.

131. Hernández blázquez M, Cruzado JA. A longitudinal study on anxiety, depressive and adjustment disorder, suicide ideation and symptoms of emotional distress in patients with cancer undergoing radiotherapy. J Psychosom Res. 2016;87:14-21.

132. Khalil A, Faheem M, Fahim A, et al. Prevalence of Depression and Anxiety amongst Cancer Patients in a Hospital Setting: A Cross-Sectional Study. Psychiatry J. 2016.

133. Sveistrup J, Mortensen OS, Bjørner JB, Engelholm SA, Munck af rosenschöld P, Petersen PM. Prospective assessment of the quality of life before, during and after image guided intensity modulated radiotherapy for prostate cancer. Radiat Oncol. 2016;11(1):117.

134. Cui W, Bennett AW, Zhang P, et al. A non-human primate model of radiation-induced cachexia. Sci Rep. 2016;6:23612.

135. Dobroś K, Hajto-bryk J, Wróblewska M, Zarzecka J. Radiation-induced caries as the late effect of radiation therapy in the head and neck region. Contemp Oncol (Pozn). 2016;20(4):287-90.

136. Maesschalck T, Dulguerov N, Caparrotti F, et al. Comparison of the incidence of osteoradionecrosis with conventional radiotherapy and intensity-modulated radiotherapy. Head Neck. 2016;38(11):1695-1702.

137. Ship JA, Eisbruch A, D'hondt E, Jones RE. Parotid sparing study in head and neck cancer patients receiving bilateral radiation therapy: one-year results. J Dent Res. 1997;76(3):807-13.

138. Grundmann O, Mitchell GC, Limesand KH. Sensitivity of salivary glands to radiation: from animal models to therapies. J Dent Res. 2009;88(10):894-903.

139. Kangas M, Milross C, Taylor A, Bryant RA. A pilot randomized controlled trial of a brief early intervention for reducing posttraumatic stress disorder, anxiety and depressive symptoms in newly diagnosed head and neck cancer patients. Psychooncology. 2013;22(7):1665-73.

140. Hofman M, Ryan JL, Figueroa-moseley CD, Jean-pierre P, Morrow GR. Cancer-related fatigue: the scale of the problem. Oncologist. 2007;12 Suppl 1:4-10.

141. Ahuja D, Bharati SJ, Gupta N, Kumar R, Bhatnagar S. Possible role of aprepitant for intractable nausea and vomiting following whole brain radiotherapy-a case report. Ann Palliat Med. 2016;5(4):315-318.

142. Spotten L, Corish C, Lorton C, et al. Subjective taste and smell changes in treatment-naive people with solid tumours. Support Care Cancer. 2016;24(7):3201-8.

143. Graner DE, Foote RL, Kasperbauer JL, et al. Swallow function in patients before and after intra-arterial chemoradiation. Laryngoscope. 2003;113(3):573-9.

144. Peters E, Mendoza schulz L, Reuss-borst M. Quality of life after cancer-How the extent of impairment is influenced by patient characteristics. BMC Cancer. 2016;16(1):787.

145. Oates JE, Clark JR, Read J, et al. Prospective evaluation of quality of life and nutrition before and after treatment for nasopharyngeal carcinoma. Arch Otolaryngol Head Neck Surg. 2007;133(6):533-40.

146. Le W, Huang S, Gui Y, et al. Assessment of numerical chromosomal abnormalities of the sperms before and after radiotherapy in seminoma patient. Int J Clin Exp Med. 2014;7(3):703-8.

147. Brignardello E, Felicetti F, Castiglione A, et al. Gonadal status in long-term male survivors of childhood cancer. J Cancer Res Clin Oncol. 2016;142(5):1127-32.

148. Apperley JF, Reddy N. Mechanism and management of treatment-related gonadal failure in recipients of high dose chemoradiotherapy. Blood Rev. 1995;9(2):93-116.

149. Zhou W, Yang X, Dai Y, Wu Q, He G, Yin G. Survey of cervical cancer survivors regarding quality of life and sexual function. J Cancer Res Ther. 2016;12(2):938-44.

150. Bandak M, Jørgensen N, Juul A, et al. Testosterone deficiency in testicular cancer survivors - a systematic review and meta-analysis. Andrology. 2016;4(3):382-8.

151. Resnick MJ, Koyama T, Fan KH, et al. Long-term functional outcomes after treatment for localized prostate cancer. N Engl J Med. 2013;368(5):436-45.

152. Hojan K, Milecki P. Opportunities for rehabilitation of patients with radiation fibrosis syndrome. Rep Pract Oncol Radiother. 2014;19(1):1-6.

153. Kopp H. Radiation damage caused by shoe-fitting fluoroscope. Br Med J. 1957;2(5057):1344-5.

154. Knobf MT, Sun Y. A longitudinal study of symptoms and self-care activities in women treated with primary radiotherapy for breast cancer. Cancer Nurs. 2005;28(3):210-8.

155. Piccin O, Sorrenti G, Milano F. Two Cases of Severe Obstructive Sleep Apnea Induced by Neck Radiotherapy Treated with an Oral Device. J Maxillofac Oral Surg. 2016;15(3):400-403.

156. Bergström L, Ward EC, Finizia C. Voice rehabilitation for laryngeal cancer patients: Functional outcomes and patient perceptions. Laryngoscope. 2016;126(9):2029-35.

157. Alba JR, Basterra J, Ferrer JC, Santonja F, Zapater E. Hypothyroidism in patients treated with radiotherapy for head and neck carcinoma: standardised long-term follow-up study. J Laryngol Otol. 2016;130(5):478-81.

158. Rayome RG, King C, King T. Patient with nocturnal enuresis and stress incontinence after previous

hysterectomy and radiation therapy for cervical cancer. J Wound Ostomy Continence Nurs. 1995;22(1):64-7.

159. Faithfull S. 'Just grin and bear it and hope that it will go away': coping with urinary symptoms from pelvic radiotherapy. Eur J Cancer Care (Engl). 1995;4(4):158-65.

160. Kollmorgen CF, Meagher AP, Wolff BG, Pemberton JH, Martenson JA, Illstrup DM. The long-term effect of adjuvant postoperative chemoradiotherapy for rectal carcinoma on bowel function. Ann Surg. 1994;220(5):676-82.

161. Müller K, Meineke V. Radiation-induced mast cell mediators differentially modulate chemokine release from dermal fibroblasts. J Dermatol Sci. 2011;61(3):199-205.

162. Müller K, Gilbertz KP, Meineke V. Serotonin and ionizing radiation synergistically affect proliferation and adhesion molecule expression of malignant melanoma cells. J Dermatol Sci. 2012;68(2):89-98.

163. Sohun M, Shen H. The implication and potential applications of high-mobility group box 1 protein in breast cancer. Ann Transl Med. 2016;4(11):217.

164. Azzam EI, Jay-gerin JP, Pain D. Ionizing radiation-induced metabolic oxidative stress and prolonged cell injury. Cancer Lett. 2012;327(1-2):48-60.

165. Bravatà V, Minafra L, Russo G, et al. High-dose Ionizing Radiation Regulates Gene Expression Changes in the MCF7 Breast Cancer Cell Line. Anticancer Res. 2015;35(5):2577-91.

166. Constine LS, Rubin P, Woolf PD, Doane K, Lush CM. Hyperprolactinemia and hypothyroidism following cytotoxic therapy for central nervous system malignancies. J Clin Oncol. 1987;5(11):1841-51.

167. Judge JL, Owens KM, Pollock SJ, et al. Ionizing radiation induces myofibroblast differentiation via lactate dehydrogenase. Am J Physiol Lung Cell Mol Physiol. 2015;309(8):879-887.

EARLY DETECTION, EARLY CURE?

1. World Health Organization. (2017). Cancer Fact Sheet. Available: http://www.who.int/mediacentre/factsheets/fs297/en. [February 3rd, 2017].

2. American Cancer Society. Breast Cancer Early Detection and Diagnosis. Available: https://www.cancer.org/cancer/breast-cancer/screening-tests-and-early-detection.html. [January 15th, 2017].

3. Kuriyama M, Wang MC, Lee CL, et al. Multiple marker evaluation in human prostate cancer with the use of tissue-specific antigens. J Natl Cancer Inst. 1982;68(1):99-105.

4. Stamey TA, Caldwell M, Mcneal JE, Nolley R, Hemenez M, Downs J. The prostate specific antigen era in the United States is over for prostate cancer: what happened in the last 20 years?. J Urol. 2004;172(4 Pt 1):1297-301.

5. Volk RJ, Wolf AM. Grading the new US Preventive Services Task Force prostate cancer screening recommendation. JAMA. 2011;306(24):2715-6.

6. Lin K, Croswell JM, Koenig H, Lam C, Maltz A. Prostate-Specific Antigen-Based Screening for Prostate Cancer: An Evidence Update for the U.S. Preventive Services Task Force. 2011; report no. 12-05160-EF-1.

7. Andriole GL, Crawford ED, Grubb RL, et al. Prostate cancer screening in the randomized Prostate, Lung, Colorectal, and Ovarian Cancer Screening Trial: mortality results after 13 years of follow-up. J Natl Cancer Inst. 2012;104(2):125-32.

8. Wilt TJ, Brawer MK, Jones KM, et al. Radical prostatectomy versus observation for localized prostate cancer. N Engl J Med. 2012;367(3):203-13.

9. Ablin J.R. 2010. The Great Prostate Mistake. *The New York Times.* Available: http://www.nytimes.com/2010/03/10/opinion/10Ablin.html. [February 3, 2017].

10. Welch HG, Albertsen PC. Prostate cancer diagnosis and treatment after the introduction of prostate-specific antigen screening: 1986-2005. J Natl Cancer Inst. 2009;101(19):1325-9.

11. Langreth, R. 2009. The Dark Side of Prostate Cancer Screening. *Forbes.* Available: http://www.forbes.com/2009/08/31/prostate-cancer-screening-business-healthcare-prostate.html. [February 3, 2017].

12. Aizer AA, Gu X, Chen MH, et al. Cost implications and complications of overtreatment of low-risk

prostate cancer in the United States. J Natl Compr Canc Netw. 2015;13(1):61-8.

13. Seu K, Casciotti D, Bravo BFD, Chen M, Jury NJ. 2016. Are annual prostate cancer screenings necessary? Should early stage prostate cancer be treated? *National Center for Health Research.* Available: http://center4research.org/child-teen-health/general-health-and-mental-health/are-annual-prostate-cancer-screenings-necessary-should-early-stage-prostate-cancer-be-treated. [February 3, 2017].

14. Hansen NM, Ye X, Grube BJ, Giuliano AE. Manipulation of the primary breast tumor and the incidence of sentinel node metastases from invasive breast cancer. Arch Surg. 2004;139(6):634-9.

15. Hoover HC, Ketcham AS. Techniques for inhibiting tumor metastases. Cancer. 1975;35(1):5-14.

16. Mathenge EG, Dean CA, Clements D, et al. Core needle biopsy of breast cancer tumors increases distant metastases in a mouse model. Neoplasia. 2014;16(11):950-60.

17. Hobson J, Gummadidala P, Silverstrim B, et al. Acute inflammation induced by the biopsy of mouse mammary tumors promotes the development of metastasis. Breast Cancer Res Treat. 2013;139(2):391-401.

18. Rosario DJ, Lane JA, Metcalfe C, et al. Short term outcomes of prostate biopsy in men tested for cancer by prostate specific antigen: prospective evaluation within ProtecT study. BMJ. 2012;344:d7894.

19. Helfand BT, Glaser AP, Rimar K, et al. Prostate cancer diagnosis is associated with an increased risk of

erectile dysfunction after prostate biopsy. BJU Int. 2013;111(1):38-43.

20. Hwang EC, Yu HS, Jung SI, Park HJ. Infectious Complications after Prostate Biopsy: A Prospective Multicenter Prostate Biopsy Study. Urogenit Tract Infect 2016;11(1):17-24.

21. Gallina A, Suardi N, Montorsi F, et al. Mortality at 120 days after prostatic biopsy: a population-based study of 22,175 men. Int J Cancer. 2008;123(3):647-52.

22. Loeb S, Carter HB, Berndt SI, Ricker W, Schaeffer EM. Complications after prostate biopsy: data from SEER-Medicare. J Urol. 2011;186(5):1830-4.

23. Resnick MJ, Koyama T, Fan KH, Albertsen PC, Goodman M, Hamilton AS, Hoffman RM, Potosky AL, Stanford JL, Stroup AM, Van Horn RL, Penson DF. Long-term functional outcomes after treatment for localized prostate cancer. N Engl J Med 2013;368(5):436-45. doi: 10.1056/NEJMoa1209978. Urol Oncol. 2013;32(4):513-4.

24. Lamplugh M, Gilmore P, Quinlan T, Cornford P. PSA testing: are patients aware of what lies ahead?. Ann R Coll Surg Engl. 2006;88(3):284-8.

25. Justman S. Uninformed consent: mass screening for prostate cancer. Bioethics. 2012;26(3):143-8.

26. Retsky M, Demicheli R, Hrushesky W, Baum M, Gukas I. Surgery triggers outgrowth of latent distant disease in breast cancer: an inconvenient truth?. Cancers (Basel). 2010;2(2):305-37.

27. Miller AB, To T, Baines CJ, Wall C. The Canadian National Breast Screening Study-1: breast cancer

mortality after 11 to 16 years of follow-up. A randomized screening trial of mammography in women age 40 to 49 years. Ann Intern Med. 2002;137(5 Part 1):305-12.

28. Miller AB, To T, Baines CJ, Wall C. Canadian National Breast Screening Study-2: 13-year results of a randomized trial in women aged 50-59 years. J Natl Cancer Inst. 2000;92(18):1490-9.

29. Miller AB, Wall C, Baines CJ, Sun P, To T, Narod SA. Twenty five year follow-up for breast cancer incidence and mortality of the Canadian National Breast Screening Study: randomised screening trial. BMJ. 2014;348:g366.

30. Von euler-chelpin M, Kuchiki M, Vejborg I. Increased risk of breast cancer in women with false-positive test: the role of misclassification. Cancer Epidemiol. 2014;38(5):619-22.

31. Christiansen CL, Wang F, Barton MB, et al. Predicting the cumulative risk of false-positive mammograms. J Natl Cancer Inst. 2000;92(20):1657-66.

32. Bleyer A, Welch HG. Effect of three decades of screening mammography on breast-cancer incidence. N Engl J Med. 2012;367(21):1998-2005.

33. Kornguth PJ, Keefe FJ, Conaway MR. Pain during mammography: characteristics and relationship to demographic and medical variables. Pain. 1996;66(2-3):187-94.

34. Van netten JP, Cann SA, Hall JG. Mammography controversies: time for informed consent?. J Natl Cancer Inst. 1997;89(15):1164-5.

35. Epstein SE. 2002. Mammography Doesn't Come Without Risk. *Los Angeles Times.* Available: http://articles.latimes.com/2002/feb/25/opinion/oe-epstein25 [February 3, 2017].

36. Eon3. Sept 29, 2015. *Pt. 1 – Medical X-rays and Breast Cancer – Dr. John Gofman.* Available: https://www.youtube.com/watch?v=AzW0zIjKcmE [February 3, 2017].

37. Modan B, Ron E, Werner A. Thyroid cancer following scalp irradiation. Radiology. 1977;123(3):741-4.

38. Boice JD, Preston D, Davis FG, Monson RR. Frequent chest X-ray fluoroscopy and breast cancer incidence among tuberculosis patients in Massachusetts. Radiat Res. 1991;125(2):214-22.

39. Baverstock KF, Vennart J. A note on radium body content and breast cancer in U.K. radium luminisers. Health Phys. 1983;44 Suppl 1:575-7.

40. Boice JD, Monson RR. Breast cancer in women after repeated fluoroscopic examinations of the chest. J Natl Cancer Inst. 1977;59(3):823-32.

41. Boice JD, Rosenstein M, Trout ED. Estimation of breast doses and breast cancer risk associated with repeated fluoroscopic chest examinations of women with tuberculosis. Radiat Res. 1978;73(2):373-90.

42. Harvey EB, Boice JD, Honeyman M, Flannery JT. Prenatal x-ray exposure and childhood cancer in twins. N Engl J Med. 1985;312(9):541-5.

43. Hoffman DA, Lonstein JE, Morin MM, Visscher W, Harris BS, Boice JD. Breast cancer in women with

scoliosis exposed to multiple diagnostic x rays. J Natl Cancer Inst. 1989;81(17):1307-12.

44. Miller AB, Howe GR, Sherman GJ, et al. Mortality from breast cancer after irradiation during fluoroscopic examinations in patients being treated for tuberculosis. N Engl J Med. 1989;321(19):1285-9.

45. Modan B, Chetrit A, Alfandary E, Katz L. Increased risk of breast cancer after low-dose irradiation. Lancet. 1989;1(8639):629-31.

46. Baverstock KF, Papworth D, Vennart J. Risks of radiation at low dose rates. Lancet. 1981;1(8217):430-3.

47. Myrden JA, Hiltz JE. Breast cancer following multiple fluoroscopies during artificial pneumothorax treatment of pulmonary tuberculosis. Can Med Assoc J. 1969;100(22):1032-4.

48. Giles D, Hewitt D, Stewart A, Webb J. Malignant disease in childhood and diagnostic irradiation in utero. Lancet. 1956;271(6940):447.

49. Stewart A, Webb J, Hewitt D. A survey of childhood malignancies. Br Med J. 1958;1(5086):1495-508.

50. Stewart A, Kneale GW. Radiation dose effects in relation to obstetric x-rays and childhood cancers. Lancet. 1970;1(7658):1185-8.

51. Andrieu N, Easton DF, Chang-claude J, et al. Effect of chest X-rays on the risk of breast cancer among BRCA1/2 mutation carriers in the international BRCA1/2 carrier cohort study: a report from the EMBRACE, GENEPSO, GEO-HEBON, and IBCCS

Collaborators' Group. J Clin Oncol. 2006;24(21):3361-6.

52. Giles D, Hewitt D, Stewart A, Webb J. Malignant disease in childhood and diagnostic irradiation in utero. Lancet. 1956;271(6940):447.

53. Bartley K, Metayer C, Selvin S, Ducore J, Buffler P. Diagnostic X-rays and risk of childhood leukaemia. Int J Epidemiol. 2010;39(6):1628-37.

54. Giovanetti A, Deshpande T, Basso E. Persistence of genetic damage in mice exposed to low dose of X rays. Int J Radiat Biol. 2008;84(3):227-35.

55. Goto H, Watanabe T, Miyao M, Fukuda H, Sato Y, Oshida Y. Cancer mortality among atomic bomb survivors exposed as children. Environ Health Prev Med. 2012;17(3):228-34.

56. Watanabe T, Miyao M, Honda R, Yamada Y. Hiroshima survivors exposed to very low doses of A-bomb primary radiation showed a high risk for cancers. Environ Health Prev Med. 2008;13(5):264-70.

57. Schmitz-feuerhake I, Busby C, Pflugbeil S. Genetic radiation risks: a neglected topic in the low dose debate. Environ Health Toxicol. 2016;31:e2016001.

58. Burlakova, E.B. 2000. *Low Doses of Radiation: Are They Dangerous?* Nova Science Pub Inc. 378 pps.

59. Busby, C. (2016). The 'Genetics' letter, the Euratom suicide clause, and the death of the nuclear industry. *The Ecologist.* Available: http://www.theecologist.org/campaigning/2988466/t he_genetics_letter_the_euratom_suicide_clause_and_t

he_death_of_the_nuclear_industry.html. [February 3, 2017].

60. R.W. Gibson, M.D., National Enquirer, December 5, 1971, 11) as reported in the book Indicted!: The People Vs the Medical & Drug Cartel by James Henderson. (2009).

61. Leslie Freeman, ed., Nuclear Witnesses: Insiders Speak Out, New York: Norton, 1982, p.27.

62. Peat, R. (2011). Radiation and growth: Incoherent imprinting from inappropriate irradiation. Available: http://raypeat.com/pdf/Radiation-and-Growth-January-2011.pdf. [February 3, 2017].

63. Jacobson JA, Danforth DN, Cowan KH, et al. Ten-year results of a comparison of conservation with mastectomy in the treatment of stage I and II breast cancer. N Engl J Med. 1995;332(14):907-11.

64. Vila J, Gandini S, Gentilini O. Overall survival according to type of surgery in young (≤40 years) early breast cancer patients: A systematic meta-analysis comparing breast-conserving surgery versus mastectomy. Breast. 2015;24(3):175-81.

65. Kummerow KL, Du L, Penson DF, Shyr Y, Hooks MA. Nationwide trends in mastectomy for early-stage breast cancer. JAMA Surg. 2015;150(1):9-16.

66. Sabel MS, Dal cin S. Trends in Media Reports of Celebrities' Breast Cancer Treatment Decisions. Ann Surg Oncol. 2016;23(9):2795-801.

67. Polivy J. Psychological effects of mastectomy on a woman's feminine self-concept. J Nerv Ment Dis. 1977;164(2):77-87.

68. José Manuel García Arroyo and María Luisa Domínguez López, "Psychological Problems Derived from Mastectomy: A Qualitative Study," International Journal of Surgical Oncology, vol. 2011, Article ID 132461, 8 pages, 2011.

69. Margolis G, Goodman RL, Rubin A. Psychological effects of breast-conserving cancer treatment and mastectomy. Psychosomatics. 1990;31(1):33-9.

70. Le GM, O'malley CD, Glaser SL, et al. Breast implants following mastectomy in women with early-stage breast cancer: prevalence and impact on survival. Breast Cancer Res. 2005;7(2):184-193.

THE BATTLE FOR TRUTH

1. Brown, J. (2006). *Judge Finds Big Tobacco Guilty of Racketeering, Conspiracy.* [Online]. Available: http://www.pbs.org/newshour/bb/law-july-dec06-smoking_08-18. [February 3, 2017].

2. Proctor RN. The history of the discovery of the cigarette-lung cancer link: evidentiary traditions, corporate denial, global toll. Tob Control. 2012;21(2):87-91.

3. Levin M. (2006). *Big Tobacco is Guilty of Conspiracy.* Los Angeles Times. [Online]. Available: http://articles.latimes.com/2006/aug/18/nation/na-smoke18.[February 5, 2017].

4. Piff PK, Stancato DM, Côté S, Mendoza-denton R, Keltner D. Higher social class predicts increased unethical behavior. Proc Natl Acad Sci USA. 2012;109(11):4086-91.

5. Côté S, Piff PK, Willer R. For whom do the ends justify the means? Social class and utilitarian moral judgment. J Pers Soc Psychol. 2013;104(3):490-503.

6. Dubois D, Rucker DD, Galinsky AD. Social class, power, and selfishness: when and why upper and lower class individuals behave unethically. J Pers Soc Psychol. 2015;108(3):436-49.

7. Bowers, S. (2012). *Global profits for tobacco trade total $35bn as smoking deaths top 6 million.* The Guardian. [Online].   Available: https://www.theguardian.com/business/2012/mar/2 2/tobacco-profits-deaths-6-million.[February 5, 2017].

8. Howard DH, Bach PB, Berndt ER, Conti RM. Pricing in the Market for Anticancer Drugs. J Econ Perspec. 2015; 29(1):139-162.

9. (2016). *These New Cancer Drugs Are Helping Patients Live Years Longer.* Fortune. [Online]. Available: http://fortune.com/2016/05/19/cancer-drugs-keytruda-opdivo.[February 5, 2017].

10. Bach PB, Conti RM, Muller RJ, Schnorr GC, Saltz LB. Overspending driven by oversized single dose vials of cancer drugs. BMJ. 2016;352:i788.

11. Tobey Jr, C. *Charles Tobey Jr. Reports On Cancer and The Venal Medical Conspiracy.* Whale.to. [Online]. Available: http://www.whale.to/p/tobey.html. [February 5, 2017].

12. Hon. William Langer, US Congressional Record, August 3, 1953, p. A 5352. Available: http://www.newmediaexplorer.org/chris/Fitzgerald% 20Report%201953.pdf.[February 5, 2017].

13. Drope J, Chapman S. Tobacco industry efforts at discrediting scientific knowledge of environmental tobacco smoke: a review of internal industry documents. J Epidemiol Community Health. 2001;55(8):588-94.

14. Olsen AH, Njor SH, Vejborg I, et al. Breast cancer mortality in Copenhagen after introduction of mammography screening: cohort study. BMJ. 2005;330(7485):220.

15. Jørgensen KJ, Zahl PH, Gøtzsche PC. Breast cancer mortality in organised mammography screening in Denmark: comparative study. BMJ. 2010;340:c1241.

16. Benjamin DJ. The efficacy of surgical treatment of breast cancer. Med Hypotheses. 1996;47(5):389-97.

17. Castillo, M. (2012). *Bra aims to detect breast cancer before mammogram.* CBS News. [Online]. Available: http://www.cbsnews.com/news/bra-aims-to-detect-breast-cancer-before-mammogram/.[February 5, 2017].

18. Fowler, E. (2015). *New Study Finds Huge Price Differences For Mammograms & Other Critical Women's Health Procedures in the 30 Largest U.S. Cities.* Castlight Health. [Online]. Available: http://www.castlighthealth.com/press-releases/new-study-finds-huge-price-differences-for-mammograms-other-critical-womens-health-procedures-in-the-30-largest-u-s-cities.[February 5, 2017].

19. Effects of radiotherapy and surgery in early breast cancer. An overview of the randomized trials. Early Breast Cancer Trialists' Collaborative Group. N Engl J Med. 1995;333(22):1444-55.

20. Adjuvant radiotherapy for rectal cancer: a systematic overview of 8,507 patients from 22 randomised trials. Lancet. 2001;358(9290):1291-304.

21. Clarke M, Collins R, Darby S, et al. Effects of radiotherapy and of differences in the extent of surgery for early breast cancer on local recurrence and 15-year survival: an overview of the randomised trials. Lancet. 2005;366(9503):2087-106.

22. Brown BW, Brauner C, Minnotte MC. Noncancer deaths in white adult cancer patients. J Natl Cancer Inst. 1993;85(12):979-87.

23. (2012). *U.S. Preventive Servies Task Force Ruling on PSA Testing a Major Blow to Men's Health.* [Online]. Available: http://pintsforprostates.org/u-s-preventive-services-task-force-ruling-on-psa-testing-a-major-blow-to-mens-health/.[February 5, 2017].

24. Public and Professional Reactions to U.S. Preventive Services Task Force Recommendations on PSA Screening. Dr. Catalona. [Online]. Available: http://www.drcatalona.com/quest/Winter2011/articl e2.html.[February 5, 2017].

25. Burne, J. (2012). *The expert branded a woman hater for saying breast cancer screening ruins lives.* [Online].Available: http://www.dailymail.co.uk/health/article-2120750/The-expert-branded-woman-hater-saying-breast-cancer-screening-ruins-lives.html#ixzz1qOQwifwi.[February 5, 2017].

26. Gøtzsche PC, Olsen O. Is screening for breast cancer with mammography justifiable?. Lancet. 2000;355(9198):129-34.

27. Nikiforov YE, Seethala RR, Tallini G, et al. Nomenclature Revision for Encapsulated Follicular Variant of Papillary Thyroid Carcinoma: A Paradigm Shift to Reduce Overtreatment of Indolent Tumors. JAMA Oncol. 2016;2(8):1023-9.

28. Kolata, G. (2016). *It's Not Cancer: Doctors Reclassify a Thyroid Tumor.* [Online]. Available: https://www.nytimes.com/2016/04/15/health/thyroid-tumor-cancer-reclassification.html?_r=2.[February 5, 2017].

29. Ablin, R.J. and Piana R. 2014. The Great Prostate Hoax: How Big Medicine Hijacked the PSA Test and Caused a Public Health Disaster. St. Martin's Press., New York, NY.

30. Johansson JE, Adami HO, Andersson SO, Bergström R, Holmberg L, Krusemo UB. High 10-year survival rate in patients with early, untreated prostatic cancer. JAMA. 1992;267(16):2191-6.

31. Schweizer MT, Antonarakis ES, Wang H, et al. Effect of bipolar androgen therapy for asymptomatic men with castration-resistant prostate cancer: results from a pilot clinical study. Sci Transl Med. 2015;7(269).

32. Stattin P, Holmberg E, Johansson JE, et al. Outcomes in localized prostate cancer: National Prostate Cancer Register of Sweden follow-up study. J Natl Cancer Inst. 2010;102(13):950-8.

33. Cooperberg MR, Ramakrishna NR, Duff SB, et al. Primary treatments for clinically localised prostate cancer: a comprehensive lifetime cost-utility analysis. BJU Int. 2013;111(3):437-50.

34. American Cancer Society. (2015). *Breast Carcinoma in Situ Cancer Facts & Figures.* [Online]. Available: https://www.cancer.org/content/dam/cancer-org/research/cancer-facts-and-statistics/annual-cancer-facts-and-figures/2015/special-section-breast-carcinoma-in-situ-cancer-facts-and-figures-2015.pdf.[February 5, 2017].

35. Kerlikowske K. Epidemiology of ductal carcinoma in situ. J Natl Cancer Inst Monographs. 2010;2010(41):139-41.

36. Demicheli R, Retsky MW, Hrushesky WJ, Baum M, Gukas ID. The effects of surgery on tumor growth: a century of investigations. Ann Oncol. 2008;19(11):1821-8.

37. Narod SA, Iqbal J, Giannakeas V, Sopik V, Sun P. Breast Cancer Mortality After a Diagnosis of Ductal Carcinoma In Situ. JAMA Oncol. 2015;1(7):888-96.

38. Esserman L, Yau C. Rethinking the Standard for Ductal Carcinoma In Situ Treatment. JAMA Oncol. 2015;1(7):881-3.

39. Drew PJ, Turnbull LW, Kerin MJ, Carleton PJ, Fox JN. Multicentricity and recurrence of breast cancer. Lancet. 1997;349(9046):208-9.

40. Penson DF, Albertsen PC. *The Natural History of Prostate Cancer.* Springer Netherlands. 2007. Available: http://link.springer.com/chapter/10.1007/978-1-4020-5847-9_2 [February 5, 2017].

41. Le Dran HF. Traite des operations de chirurgie. Paris: C. Osmont; 1742.

42. Larsen SU, Rose C. [Spontaneous remission of breast cancer. A literature review]. Ugeskr Laeg. 1999;161(26):4001-4.

43. Monzen Y, Nakahara M, Nishisaka T. Spontaneous regression of primary malignant lymphoma of the prostate. Case Rep Urol. 2013;2013:363072.

44. Banihani MN, Al manasra AR. Spontaneous regression in alveolar soft part sarcoma: case report and literature review. World J Surg Oncol. 2009;7:53.

45. Tanaka K, Hamada T, Takasaki H, Yokoyama S. Spontaneous regression of mediastinal seminoma. OAI. 1989.

46. Printz C. Spontaneous Regression of Melanoma May Offer Insight Into Cancer Immunology. J Nat Can Inst. 2001; 93 (14): 1047-1048.

47. Papac RJ. Spontaneous regression of cancer: possible mechanisms. In Vivo. 1998;12(6):571-8.

48. Ogawa D, Uemura N, Sasaki N, et al. Spontaneous regression of malignant lymphoma of the stomach. J Med. 1998;29(5-6):381-93.

49. Bir AS, Fora AA, Levea C, Fakih MG. Spontaneous regression of colorectal cancer metastatic to retroperitoneal lymph nodes. Anticancer Res. 2009;29(2):465-8.

50. Stefani C, Liverani CA, Bianco V, et al. Spontaneous regression of low-grade cervical intraepithelial lesions is positively improved by topical bovine colostrum preparations (GINEDIE®). A multicentre, observational, italian pilot study. Eur Rev Med Pharmacol Sci. 2014;18(5):728-33.

51. Iwanaga T. [Studies on cases of spontaneous regression of cancer in Japan in 2011, and of hepatic carcinoma, lung cancer and pulmonary metastases in the world between 2006 and 2011]. Gan To Kagaku Ryoho. 2013;40(11):1475-87.

52. Davis T, Doyle H, Tobias V, Ellison DW, Ziegler DS. Case Report of Spontaneous Resolution of a Congenital Glioblastoma. Pediatrics. 2016;137(4).

53. Isobe Y, Aritaka N, Sasaki M, Oshimi K, Sugimoto K. Spontaneous regression of natural killer cell lymphoma. J Clin Pathol. 2009;62(7):647-50.

54. Crisci A, Corsale I, Abrami F, et al. [Spontaneous regression of lung metastases from renal cell carcinoma: the importance of immunogenetic factors and a review of the literature]. Minerva Urol Nefrol. 2008;60(2):123-35.

55. Bir AS, Fora AA, Levea C, Fakih MG. Spontaneous regression of colorectal cancer metastatic to retroperitoneal lymph nodes. Anticancer Res. 2009;29(2):465-8.

56. Paredes BE. [Regression in malignant melanoma. Definition, etiopathogenesis, morphology and differential diagnosis]. Pathologe. 2007;28(6):453-63.

57. Khar A, Muralikrishna K, Varalakshmi C. High intratumoural level of cytokines mediates efficient regression of a rat histiocytoma. Clin Exp Immunol. 1997;110(1):127-31.

58. Wong DA, Bishop GA, Lowes MA, Cooke B, Barnetson RS, Halliday GM. Cytokine profiles in spontaneously regressing basal cell carcinomas. Br J Dermatol. 2000;143(1):91-8.

59. Mueller N. Overview of the epidemiology of malignancy in immune deficiency. J Acquir Immune Defic Syndr. 1999;21 Suppl 1:S5-10.

60. Saleh F, Renno W, Klepacek I, et al. Direct evidence on the immune-mediated spontaneous regression of human cancer: an incentive for pharmaceutical companies to develop a novel anti-cancer vaccine. Curr Pharm Des. 2005;11(27):3531-43.

61. Schilder H, de Vries MJ, Goodkin K, Antoni M. Psychological Changes Preceding Spontaneous Remission of Cancer. Clinical Case Studies. 2004; 3(4):288-312.

62. Oliver RT, Nethersell AB, Bottomley JM. Unexplained spontaneous regression and alpha-interferon as treatment for metastatic renal carcinoma. Br J Urol. 1989;63(2):128-31.

63. Sroujieh AS. Spontaneous regression of intestinal malignant melanoma from an occult primary site. Cancer. 1988;62(6):1247-50.

64. Drobyski WR, Qazi R. Spontaneous regression in non-Hodgkin's lymphoma: clinical and pathogenetic considerations. Am J Hematol. 1989;31(2):138-41.

65. Horning SJ, Rosenberg SA. The natural history of initially untreated low-grade non-Hodgkin's lymphomas. N Engl J Med. 1984;311(23):1471-5.

66. Zahl PH, Maehlen J, Welch HG. The natural history of invasive breast cancers detected by screening mammography. Arch Intern Med. 2008;168(21):2311-6.

67. Barnetson RS, Halliday GM. Regression in skin tumours: a common phenomenon. Australas J Dermatol. 1997;38 Suppl 1:S63-5.

68. Zahl PH, Gøtzsche PC, Mæhlen J. Natural history of breast cancers detected in the Swedish mammography screening programme: a cohort study. Lancet Oncol. 2011;12(12):1118-24.

69. Miller AB, To T, Baines CJ, Wall C. The Canadian National Breast Screening Study-1: breast cancer mortality after 11 to 16 years of follow-up. A randomized screening trial of mammography in women age 40 to 49 years. Ann Intern Med. 2002;137(5 Part 1):305-12.

70. Miller AB, Wall C, Baines CJ, Sun P, To T, Narod SA. Twenty five year follow-up for breast cancer incidence and mortality of the Canadian National Breast Screening Study: randomised screening trial. BMJ. 2014;348.

71. Andersson I, Aspegren K, Janzon L, et al. Mammographic screening and mortality from breast cancer: the Malmö mammographic screening trial. BMJ. 1988;297(6654):943-8.

72. Fox MS. On the Diagnosis and Treatment of Breast Cancer. JAMA. 1979;241(5):489-494.

73. Jones HB. Demographic consideration of the cancer problem. Trans N Y Acad Sci. 1956;18(4):298-333.

74. Rubinow DR, Roca CA, Schmidt PJ, et al. Testosterone suppression of CRH-stimulated cortisol in men. Neuropsychopharmacology. 2005;30(10):1906-12.

75. Buchanan KL, Evans MR, Goldsmith AR, Bryant DM, Rowe LV. Testosterone influences basal metabolic rate in male house sparrows: a new cost of dominance signalling?. Proc Biol Sci. 2001;268(1474):1337-44.

76. Hofling M, Hirschberg AL, Skoog L, Tani E, Hägerström T, Von schoultz B. Testosterone inhibits estrogen/progestogen-induced breast cell proliferation in postmenopausal women. Menopause. 2007;14(2):183-90.

77. Dicker A, Rydén M, Näslund E, et al. Effect of testosterone on lipolysis in human pre-adipocytes from different fat depots. Diabetologia. 2004;47(3):420-8.

78. Hanin L, Zaider M. Effects of Surgery and Chemotherapy on Metastatic Progression of Prostate Cancer: Evidence from the Natural History of the Disease Reconstructed through Mathematical Modeling. Cancers (Basel). 2011;3(3):3632-60.

79. Periyakoil VS, Neri E, Fong A, Kraemer H. Do unto others: doctors' personal end-of-life resuscitation preferences and their attitudes toward advance directives. PLoS ONE. 2014;9(5).

INDEX

Abel, Ulrich, 38, 39

Ablin, Richard, 72-73, 75, 101,

Agnew, Hayes, 33

Allison, Wade, 54

American Cancer Society, 11, 72, 88, 107

Apoptosis, 61

Atomic Energy Commission, 84

Biopsy, 23, 63, 73, 76-77, 86,

Breast cancer, 40-41, 54-56, 59, 62, 64, 72, 78-81, 85-87, 94-96, 98, 101-102, 104, 106-107

Bross, Irwin, 84

Brunschwig, Alexander, 17

Burk, Dean, 88

Burlakova, EB, 82

Busby, Chris, 83

Caisse, Renee, 3, 91

Cancer: Principles and Practise of Oncology, 24

Cancer research, 28, 55, 93

Cancer surgery, 14-16, 22-24, 29-30, 33, 56, 95

hemicorporectomy, 15, 17

the commando, 15-16

the whipple, 15-16

total exenteration, 15-17

Carcinogenesis, 32, 61

Cell phones, 53, 62

evidence they cause cancer, 62

Chemotherapy, 3-4, 35, 38-49, 58, 66-67, 70, 86, 91, 105, 107, 109, 111,

side effects of, 41

Chernobyl nuclear disaster, 53-54

Cole, Warren, 23

Conspiracy, 89, 93

Coronary artery bypass, 20-22

Davita, Vincent J, 24

Der Spiegel, 38

d'Etoilles, Leroy, 22

Early detection, 71-72, 87-88, 95-96

Epstein, Samuel, 80

Einstein, Albert, 10

Esserman, Laura, 101

Fisher, Bernard, 55
Fitzgerald Jr, Benedict F, 92-93
Fox, Maurice, 106-107
Gerson, Max, 37
Gibson, Robert W, 84
Gofman, John, 84-85
Gonzales, Nicholas, 37
Gotzsche, Peter, 97-98, 102
Hamer, Ryke Geerd, 49
Harris, Ian, 18-20
Hippocrates, 108
Hospitals,
memorial sloan-kettering, 14-15
Milton Keynes hospiral, 40
women's hospital, 15
Hyman, Mark, 20
Inflammation, 32, 37, 43, 45, 61, 66
Ionizing radiation, 51-52, 60, 62, 80, 82-84, 104, 110
Jerome-Parks, Scott, 63-64
Jn-Charles, Alexandra, 63-64
Jones, Hardin B, 88, 107-108

Journals,
annals of surgery, 55
annals of the New York Academy of Sciences, 23
bioelectromagnetics, 62
British medical journal, 79, 94
cancer, 41
circulation, 21
international journal of radiation biology, 82
journal of the national cancer institute, 58, 74-75, 81, 100
Lancet oncology, 40
lung cancer, 57
the American Journal of Cardiology, 21
the australasian journal of dermatology, 104
the French Academy of Science, 22
the Lancet, 20, 38, 40, 55-56, 81, 98
the New England journal of medicine, 56, 74, 77, 80, 86, 103
Kessler, David, 89
Krebiozen, 91

Krebs, Ernst T, 49

Krokowski, Ernst H, 23-24

Leape, Lucian, 19

Levin, Allen, 48

Lincoln, Robert, 92

Liponis, Mark, 20

Lockwood, Skip, 97

Lymphadenectomy, 24

Mammography, 78-80, 86-87, 94-96, 98, 104-106

Markstein, Michelle, 39

Mathe, Charles, 108

Mendelsohn, Robert, 19, 33

Metastasis, 23-24, 30, 32, 33, 76, 80, 105

Methylene blue, 61

Miller, Theodore, 17

Monteith, Stan, 91

Moss, Ralph, 14-15, 57, 70, 96

Mothersill, Carmel E, 60

National Cancer Institute, 16, 24, 55, 58, 74-75, 81, 88, 100,

National Public Radio, 36

Nickiforov, Yuri E, 99

Nixon, Alan, 49

Now and Then (Bob Madison), 40

Pall, Martin, 62

Palpation, 23

Paracelsus, 108

Peat, Raymond, 1, 53, 83,

Poison gas factory workers, 39

Prostate cancer, 72-77, 88, 97, 100-102

PSA Test, 72-78, 80, 87, 97, 105

Radiation bandwidths, extra-low frequency, 62

microwave, 62

Radiation bystander effects, 60-62

Radical mastectomy, 54-55

Radical prostatectomy, 73-74

Radioactive isotopes, 53

Radiotherapy, 4, 49, 51, 53-59, 63-70, 73, 77, 79, 86, 96, 105, 109, 111

for acne, 58-59

for Hodgkin's lymphoma, 58-59

for peptic ulcers, 58-59

for scalp ringworm, 58-59

side effects of, 64
Retsky, Michael, 24
Röntgen, Wilhelm, 52
Shoe-fitting x-ray
fluoroscopes, 52
Shulze, Richard, 88
Sims, Marion J, 14-15
Spontaneous regression,
102-104
Stamey, Thomas, 73
Sternglass, Ernest, 10
*Surgery: The Ultimate
Placebo* (Harris), 18
Surgical stress, 25-29
side effects of, 25
Tabar, Laszlo, 98
The Cancer Industry
(Moss), 14, 57
The Great Prostate Hoax
(Ablin), 72
Thyroid hormone, 28,
37, 47, 57, 69, 99, 102
The Fitzgerald report,
92-93
The Lincoln Treatment,
92
Timeless quotes, 33, 48,
70, 88, 108
Tobey Jr, Charles, 92
Tumor, 13-14, 22-24, 27-
33, 36-39, 44, 47-48,
51-52, 62, 65, 69-70,
86, 99, 102-103, 104-
105, 112
Tumor
microenvironment, 28-
29, 47, 69
adrenaline, 29-30, 47,
69
cortisol, 29, 31-32, 47,
69
epidermal growth
factor, 29-30, 48, 69
estrogen, 29, 31, 41, 47,
62, 69, 100
free radicals, 28, 30, 47,
69
high mobility group
box 1 protein, 28
histamine, 29, 31, 48,
70
interleukin-1 beta, 28,
69
interleukin-4, 38, 69
interleukin-6, 28, 47, 69
interleukin-8, 29, 47, 69
lactic acid, 29, 31, 48,
70
nitric oxide, 29, 30, 47,
61-62, 69
nuclear factor kappa
beta, 29, 32, 47, 69

prolactin, 29, 32, 47, 69
prostaglandins, 29-30,
47, 70
serotonin, 29, 31, 48,
70
tumor necrosis factor
alpha, 28, 32, 47, 69,
130
vascular endothelial
growth factor, 29, 30,
48, 69
Ultraprevention (Hyman
and Liponis), 20
Universities,
Harvard university, 19,
24, 39, 60, 107
Kuwait university, 105
McMaster university,
60
Princeton university,
10
university of Buffalo,
84
university of California,
81, 84, 88, 102, 107
university of Illinois, 23
university of
Massachusetts, 39, 92
university of oxford, 54
university of
Pittsburgh, 99

university of
Washington, 61, 62
Yale university, 36
US Preventive Services
Task Force, 74, 88, 97,
Velpeau, Alfred-
Armand-Louis-Marie,
33
Warner, Glen, 108
War on cancer, 9
Watson, James, 88
Wayman, Richard, 63
Welch, Gilbert H, 75-76
Whipple, Allen
Oldfather, 15-16
Whitaker, Julian, 70
Woolf, Steven H, 88
World Health
Organization, 11, 71
World war II, 35-36, 39,
53
X-rays, 10, 51-53, 61-63,
78, 80, 81, 83-85
Yau, Christina, 101

ABOUT THE AUTHOR

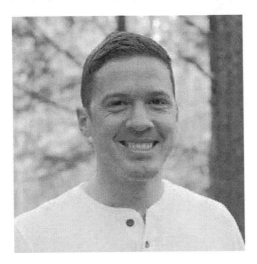

MARK SLOAN has written over 300 articles and is the author of *The Cancer Industry, Cancer: The Metabolic Disease Unravelled* and the 6x international #1 bestseller *Red Light Therapy: Miracle Medicine.* Mark lives in Ontario, Canada and his goal is to build his home from scratch, entirely off grid and live a self-sufficient, resilient and responsible life as God had intended. Mark is passionate about learning and his ultimate goal in life is to reduce the suffering in this world and to make a better place for every human being alive and for future generations.

PLEASE REVIEW THIS!

I hope you enjoyed this book and that it has given you the confidence you need to make your own health decisions. Above all, I hope it gives you hope for a brighter future.

If this book helped or entertained you in any way, all I ask in return is that you take a moment to write an honest, sincere review of this book on Amazon. It will only take a few minutes, and it will help me out more than you can imagine.

To leave a review, search "Cancer industry Mark Sloan" on Amazon to find the book page or visit the following link, then scroll down and write a couple of quick sentences:

https://amazon.com/dp/0994741847

MORE INTERNATIONAL #1 BESTSELLING BOOKS BY THE AUTHOR

- The Cancer Industry
- Cancer: The Metabolic Disease Unravelled
- Red Light Therapy: Miracle Medicine
- The Ultimate Guide to Methylene Blue: Remarkable Hope for
- Bath Bombs & Balneotherapy
- And more!

Checkout all of Mark Sloan's books by visiting the following link:
https://endalldisease.com/books

DON'T FORGET TO CLAIM YOUR 3 FREE EBOOKS AND FREE MONTHLY NEWSLETTER

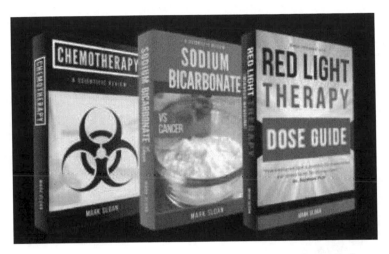

Visit the link below and enter your name and email for instant access to our ebooks. You'll also join thousands of fans and receive a free monthly email newsletter including all the latest and greatest from End All Disease.

Your Link:

WWW.ENDALLDISEASE.COM/SPECIALOFFER